# HEALTHCARE GOVERNANCE

# HEALTHCARE GOVERNANCE

## A Guide for Effective Boards

Errol L. Biggs

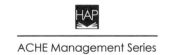

ACHE Management Series

Your board, staff, or clients may also benefit from this book's insight. For more information on quantity discounts, contact the Health Administration Press Marketing Manager at (312) 424–9470.

This publication is intended to provide accurate and authoritative information in regard to the subject matter covered. It is sold, or otherwise provided, with the understanding that the publisher is not engaged in rendering professional services. If professional advice or other expert assistance is required, the services of a competent professional should be sought.

The statements and opinions contained in this book are strictly those of the authors and do not represent the official positions of the American College of Healthcare Executives or the Foundation of the American College of Healthcare Executives.

15    14    13    12    11         5    4    3    2    1

**Library of Congress Cataloging-in-Publication Data**

Biggs, Errol L.
  Healthcare governance : a guide for effective boards / Errol L. Biggs.
    p. cm.
  ISBN 978-1-56793-419-9 (alk. paper)
  1. Hospitals--United States--Administration. 2. Health services administration--United States. I. Title.
  RA971.B574 2011
  362.11068--dc23

                    2011013845

The paper used in this publication meets the minimum requirements of American National Standard for Information Sciences—Permanence of Paper for Printed Library Materials, ANSI Z39.48-1984. ♾ ™

Acquisitions editor: Janet Davis; Project manager: Amy Carlton; Typesetting: Network Publishing Partners, Inc.

Cover illustration by Sean Kane. Copyright 2011 Sean Kane.

Found an error or a typo? We want to know! Please e-mail it to hap1@ache.org, and put "Book Error" in the subject line.

For photocopying and copyright information, please contact Copyright Clearance Center at www.copyright .com or at (978) 750–8400.

Health Administration Press
A division of the Foundation of the American
    College of Healthcare Executives
One North Franklin Street, Suite 1700
Chicago, IL 60606–3529
(312) 424–2800

*This book is dedicated to Alison Lee Biggs, truly a lovely and very smart lady, whose husband I still have the privilege to be.*

# Contents

# Preface

Being a hospital or health system board member has become more difficult during the last five years, and there appear to be even more challenges coming.

Some experts have suggested that many boards are little more than a collection of high-powered people engaged in low-level activities, rather than groups thinking and working strategically (Taylor, Chait, and Holland 1996). However, increasing numbers of boards are making concentrated efforts to function effectively and to adopt or adapt best practices from other, more successful boards.

In addition, changes in the law and other areas should cause many boards to examine how they are structured and how they conduct their business. Some of these changes include the following.

## Healthcare Reform

On March 30, 2010, President Barack Obama signed H.R. 4872, the Health Care and Education Reconciliation Act of 2010, which modified the Patient Protection and Affordable Care Act (ACA), H.R. 3590. These laws provide the foundation for changes made by Congress to the current healthcare delivery, payment, and insurance systems. The legislation may have the most significant impact on the healthcare financing system since Medicare began in 1965. The law goes into effect in phases between 2010 and 2016 with full implementation in 2020. Hospital and health systems management and boards must fully understand the components of this new legal framework.

Some aspects of the legislation may be beneficial to hospitals and health systems, such as changes to insurance markets, malpractice reform, and funding to help with high volumes of preventable readmissions. From another angle, hospitals and health systems may well be adversely affected by scheduled payment cuts. The legislation also transforms tax-exempt status and pricing transparency. How these different aspects will balance in the long run remains to be seen.

The secretary of the U.S. Department of Health and Human Services will have the power to implement much of the legislation. For example, the secretary will develop a method for assessing hospital performance in quality improvement, relating it to reimbursement. As the phrase "the secretary shall" appears more than 1,000 times in the law, boards should follow the rulemaking process closely.

## IRS Form 990

The Internal Revenue Service's (IRS) redesigned Form 990 dramatically increases the number of questions dedicated to the corporate governance of tax-exempt hospitals and health systems. This increase reflects the IRS's close scrutiny of corporate governance and the perspective that a well-governed organization is likely to be a tax-compliant organization.

The Form 990 governance emphasis contains 20 separate questions relating to the governing body and management, board policies, and disclosures.

Trustees should be aware of how many voting members on their organization's board are considered independent. The definition of "independent" indicates a director or a director's relative is not compensated by the organization or a related organization as an officer or employee; did not receive more than $10,000 a year as an independent contractor of the organization or a related organization; and did not receive a material financial benefit (more than $50,000) from the organization or a related organization. Conflicts of interest must be disclosed annually.

Other key issues include

- Reviewing the organization's Form 990 by the board or a specifically designated board committee
- Explaining "best practices" policies, including a written whistleblower policy with protections against retaliation and a document retention and destruction policy
- Justifying and structuring of salaries and perks for key employees
- Sufficiency of current policy on conflict of interest
- Examining the organization's assessment and response to community needs

Boards could use the IRS Form 990 to their advantage as a management tool, conducting a yearly audit using the form as a guide.


## American Competitiveness and Corporate Accountability Act of 2002

Commonly known as the Sarbanes-Oxley Act, this legislation mainly relates to publicly traded companies, but it also has some provisions with which several states are now asking nonprofit organizations to comply. The five main areas nonprofits should address include sections relating to

1. Audit committees being made up of independent members, including a financial expert

2. The audit committee's relationship to external auditors
3. Establishment of an audit committee charter and code of ethics
4. A requirement for executive certification of financial statements
5. Establishment of certain internal controls

## Rating Agencies

Rating agencies now ask questions of the governing board before rating a hospital's bonds. Some areas of exploration have included

- Whether the board has adopted certain sections of Sarbanes-Oxley
- Whether the audit shows any material weaknesses
- Whether audit adjustments go to the board for its review
- How the management letter from the external auditors is used

## Quality of Care

Quality, the most fundamental objective of all healthcare services, is now a public issue, no longer closely held solely by the professions. Its link to the cost of care has also moved to the forefront of the public's attention. Managing to achieve optimal, cost-effective quality and safety will continue to be a dominant governance issue for many years.

## Hospitalists

The rapid emergence of hospitalists is one example of a significant change in the organization of hospital practice, and it has implications for the financial and quality relationships between the hospital and individual physicians. This change will undoubtedly alter the role of the traditional medical staff, which is already declining and becoming more disorganized as physicians increasingly identify with medical groups and specialty associations. How the board relates to these developments while maintaining responsibility for quality and safety will be the issue.

## Other Challenges for Boards

- Development of accountable care organizations resulting from the ACA
- Growing consumer demand, fueled by the Internet, for information and accountability

- The effect of the baby boomer age wave on healthcare financing and delivery
- The continued nursing shortage and a predicted physician shortage
- The growth of complementary and alternative medicine

In these turbulent times, hospitals and health systems are fortunate to still have sincere, well-meaning individuals willing to take on the formidable task of being board members. It is important to provide support for the work of both new and seasoned members as they deal with new ideas or challenges to old ones.

Although I have worked with many boards of directors throughout my career in the healthcare industry, I am continually intrigued by boards of similar health organizations from similar communities, which vary so much in their efficiency and efficacy. Certainly, no individual agrees to serve on a board to be ineffective. However, many otherwise competent individuals have never received job descriptions or an effective orientation session, and they simply don't know their roles and responsibilities as productive healthcare board members.

This book is designed to be used by both new and experienced board members. It focuses on the best practices of board structure and function and board members' responsibilities. I developed this book during the several years I spent running hospitals and later attending eight to ten management-contract hospital board meetings a month. The work has been further advanced during my subsequent years serving on boards, working and interacting with boards, teaching graduate students about governance, consulting, and doing research about boards.

The book is structured to be perused in sections—allowing the reader to go to specific areas of interest or need—or it can be considered as a whole. My goal is to present information in a format that will be helpful regardless of the expertise of anyone using it.

## Acknowledgments

I would like to thank some individuals who were very helpful in developing several areas of the book: **Sita Ananth** (director of Knowledge Services, Samueli Institute, Alexandria, Virginia); **Alison K. Biggs,** MSHA, RN; **Kenneth Bopp** (clinical professor and director, Health Management & Informatics Group, University of Missouri, Columbia); **Donna Marshall** (executive director, Colorado Business Group on Health, Denver); **Gregory Piche** (Singularity Legal and Office of the Attorney General, State of Minnesota); **Michael Pugh** (president, Verisma Systems, Inc., Pueblo, Colorado); **Larry Tyler** (president, Tyler & Company, Atlanta); **Cathy Barry-Ipema** (chief communications officer, The Joint Commission, Oakbrook

Terrace, Illinois); **Lee Seidel** (professor of Health Administration, University of New Hampshire, Durham); **Dennis Stillman** (senior lecturer, University of Washington, Seattle); and **Bruce Sullivan** (retired partner, Ernst & Young, Nashville).

—*Errol L. Biggs*
Denver, Colorado

## Reference

Taylor, B. E., R. P. Chait, and T. P. Holland. 1996. "The New Work of the Nonprofit Board." *Harvard Business Review* 74 (5): 36–46.

# CHAPTER ONE

# Basic Responsibilities of a Board and Its Members

## MAIN RESPONSIBILITIES OF THE GOVERNING BOARD

All boards, regardless of their organization's focus, share the same traits:

- Board membership is as high as one can get and still be in the organization. It is the ultimate authority.
- Boards only have authority when they meet. Unless boards are in session in person, or have arranged to meet in a conference call, they don't have authority to act. If the board's bylaws allow, an executive committee may meet and act for the board, or the board can vote on issues by mail or email. It is important for the bylaws to detail what is considered a regular board meeting, what kind of special meetings may be called, how much advance notice is required, and any other parameters that must be met for a regular or special meeting to occur.
- No one individual has authority to act for the board. A board member may be given authority by the board to complete a purchase or carry out a specific task, but only the board as a whole has the authority to take any action.
- Boards are not like Congress or the courts. They need to speak with one voice. There should be much discussion, there may be disagreements, and opinions should be expressed. But, in the end, board members need to unite behind a majority decision.
- Time is a precious commodity. Boards need to use their time efficiently because they don't have much of it.

Although an ideal board functions as a team for the good of the organization, the very nature of a board may preclude the development of teamwork:

- **Directors are not full time.** Most independent directors have full-time jobs elsewhere, and their primary focus rests with that job, not the board.
- **There is only periodic interaction.** Board members meet together for relatively short periods of time, separated by weeks or months. This makes it difficult to build continuity or develop as a team.
- **Meeting time is limited.** Boards have a limited amount of time to spend on board activities or on any one issue. Because they are not in the organization's day-to-day information loop, board members may approach their work with limited knowledge or understanding of the nuances of particular issues.
- **Unclear authority relationships may exist.** Unlike a hierarchical management structure, board members all have equal authority, adding to the ambiguity under which a board functions.
- **Lack of clarity may exist about management versus governance.** Sometimes the distinctions between management's role and the governing board's role are not exactly clear, particularly to new board members. When the board gets involved in operations, it loses its governing effectiveness.

The board's work is done in board and committee meetings, making it absolutely essential for those meetings to be effective and productive—teamwork at its best, regardless of the factors that seem designed to prevent it.

## The Board and the Organization's Mission, Vision, and Goals

While some may feel it is obvious the board runs the show, that kind of simplistic approach ignores reality. Without a knowledge of and attention to the basic components of a board's reason for being, a board may inadvertently abdicate its responsibilities.

It is the board's responsibility to map the hospital's course through the establishment and periodic review of its mission, vision, and goals. As Lewis Carroll said, "If you don't know where you are going, any road will get you there." Without a clear understanding and agreement of what the organization wants to accomplish (its mission), how it wants to accomplish the mission (its goals), and where it wants to be in the future (its vision), a board can wander countless roads, never knowing when it has accomplished something of value or even what is valued. Strategic planning (discussed later in this chapter) is a function of the board that ties these three components together.

Once the mission, vision, and goals are established and a strategic plan is developed, the board will be able to reach its decisions. However, experience has shown that board members may not always be truly aware of the hospital's mission.

The simple act of putting the mission statement at the top of the agenda for every board and committee meeting can save time and unnecessary discussion. If board members can readily see the mission statement, their course of action will be more obvious. Some agenda items may even be dispensed with quickly if it is obvious they are not part of the mission.

To focus the entire organization on the mission statement, it should also be printed clearly on the back of all business cards and at the top of agendas for any hospital-related meetings of the board, employees, medical staff, or volunteers.

## The Board and Executive Management Performance

When dealing with the hospital's staff, the board should concentrate on the only employee who reports directly to them—the chief executive officer (CEO). Although the chief operating officer, chief financial officer, chief nursing officer, medical director, and any vice presidents are important in making the organization a success, the board does not supervise or evaluate these individuals. Many boards have difficulty staying focused on the CEO, particularly in smaller communities where everyone tends to know each other. However, it is important for that focus to remain clear.

The board does not evaluate anyone but the CEO, does not hire anyone but the CEO, does not set goals and objectives for anyone but the CEO, and does not replace anyone but the CEO. The board also needs to be assured there is management depth in the organization and that succession planning and management development activities are a priority for the CEO. No organization can afford to flounder during a transition from one CEO to another.

## The Board Ensures the Quality of Patient Care

The hospital or health system board can and should delegate the design, implementation, and measurement of the quality of care to administration and staff. However, the board is legally and ultimately responsible for ensuring quality care is available and provided to patients. As such, the board needs to be comfortable the systems are in place to make that assurance, and it needs to see indicators that allow a lay board member to understand the hospital's quality compared with the quality at similar organizations (benchmarking).

There are many quality-outcome indicators, including

- hospital-acquired infections,
- surgical wound infections,
- neonatal mortality,
- inpatient mortality,
- cesarean section rate,
- unplanned readmissions to the hospital,
- unplanned returns to the operating room,
- pressure ulcers (bed sores),
- patient falls,
- nurse hours per patient day,
- patient satisfaction with pain management, and
- overall patient satisfaction.

The board, through its quality committee, should develop dashboard indicators—the ratios, numbers, or percentages that measure activity—to alert it to unacceptable quality outcomes.

Effective boards raise the importance of quality care to equal or surpass financial matters. This sends a clear message to the administration, the medical staff, the nursing staff, and others about the board's priorities. These boards strive to run hospitals and health systems that benchmark well in all areas of quality measurement.

### The Board Ensures the Organization's Financial Health

Most board members feel more comfortable reviewing financial statements than quality indicators, but financial health and high quality are intertwined. An organization rarely achieves quality if its finances are not on solid footing. Oddly, in many instances, experienced businesspeople have a different view of what financial health means in a nonprofit hospital from what it means in the for-profit sector. Some nonprofit boards think nonprofit means not too much black ink, nor too much red ink, but "pink" ink—a kind of a break-even mentality.

For this reason, the use of the term "nonprofit" may do a disservice to hospitals and health systems because it frames the mind-set of the breakeven approach. A more accurate descriptor for "nonprofit" healthcare organizations would be "tax exempt."

Regardless of the board's perspective, however, a 2009 survey of top issues confronting hospitals, completed by CEOs for the American College of Healthcare Executives (ACHE 2010), clearly shows financial challenges to be the number one issue facing hospitals and health systems.

All boards need to realize how important it is to have excess revenue over expense at least equal to the cost of capital. For example, if the board is to keep the hospital's equipment up to date or replace antiquated or inefficient buildings, it is imperative to have enough revenue/profit available to accomplish these things. As Dr. Leland Kaiser (2011), health administration faculty member from the University of Colorado Denver and nationally recognized futurist, has said, "It is virtuous to help the poor; it is not virtuous to be poor!" A hospital or health system is a business and must have excess revenue over expense to continue to provide quality care.

### Hospital Boards Assume Some Responsibility for Their Community's Health

Many hospitals and health systems are required to perform needs-assessment studies to address the health status of their communities. Board members should educate themselves about their community's rates of heart disease, cancer, teen pregnancy, and other issues. It is the board's role to determine how this should be done within the organization's resources. For example, in a city with high rates of diabetes, directors should look for ways in which the hospital can educate the community about the importance of healthy eating, exercise, and regular checkups.

### The Board Must Assume Responsibility for Itself

At a minimum, the board has a responsibility for taking care of itself, including

- establishing an effective orientation program for new members;
- conducting a self-assessment process every two to three years;
- creating a continuing education program for all members;
- subscribing to relevant periodicals, such as *Trustee*; and
- maintaining up-to-date job descriptions for all members and officers.

Job descriptions are perhaps the most important of these. If new board members receive current job descriptions from the board chair, they will be much less confused about the role of the board and their specific roles on that board.

## STRATEGIC PLANNING

In recent years, the importance of strategic planning has come to the forefront for boards of both private nonprofit and public companies. The National

Association of Corporate Directors' (NACD 2010a) survey of leading issues among public boards found strategic planning ranked first, ahead of corporate performance and financial oversight. NACD's (2010b) survey of nonprofit board members ranked strategic planning fifth out of 25 key issues. In today's turbulent environment, this similar emphasis on the importance of strategic planning is likely not a coincidence.

In the nonprofit (tax-exempt) world, as more healthcare boards evaluate their duties, boards should be actively engaged with management to ensure the appropriate development, execution, and modification of the healthcare organization's strategic plan, for several reasons:

- Healthcare reform and its many implications for hospitals, including how increased insurance coverage will affect demand for services
- Advances in medical technology
- Competition from a hospital's medical staff
- Changing reimbursement patterns as hospitals receive less from Medicare and Medicaid
- Consolidation in the healthcare industry
- Stakeholder activism, as community members become more vocal in demanding new services or more locations from their hospital

Hospitals must respond to such changes with similar speed. Hospitals and healthcare organizations without a carefully thought-out strategic plan may steer the organization in a dangerous direction with no idea where they are going.

Appropriate development of a strategic plan does not mean the board has to determine the organization's strategy or create a detailed strategic plan, as this is generally the responsibility of management.

| Management's Role in Strategic Planning | The Board's Role in Strategic Planning |
| --- | --- |
| • Develop the organization's strategy<br>• Obtain board approval for the plan<br>• Implement and communicate the strategy<br>• Routinely update the board on the plan's execution<br>• Propose changes as needed | • Evaluate the strategy proposed by management<br>• Approve the strategy<br>• Monitor its implementation<br>• Challenge assumptions and analyses as necessary<br>• Encourage changes as events require |

Management should also regularly send the board supplemental information about the organization's performance, especially trends and uncertainties that may affect the implementation of the approved strategy.

Simply put, management creates the organization's strategic plan, involving the full board in its development. With this understanding of the plan, the board will be able to intelligently approve it, monitor it, and suggest needed changes and adjustments. The board needs to review the strategic plan regularly to be comfortable with the hospital's long-term direction. The board needs to take a long-term view of the organization, its objectives, and the means to achieve them.

## BASIC LEGAL DUTIES

### The Duty of Care

The first basic legal responsibility of a board director is called *the duty of care*. This means the director must exercise appropriate diligence—doing what a reasonable person would do in the same situation with the same information—in making decisions for the organization and overseeing its management. The duty of care protects directors from liability for acting in the best interests of the organization, as long as there are rational bases for their decisions and no conflicts of interest.

To exercise the duty of care, a director can rely on information provided by others—including the organization's officers, employees, legal counsel, and committees—as long as she acts in good faith—that is, her actions are not knowingly inappropriate. In meeting their duty of care, directors must be willing to make the appropriate time commitment for regular attendance at meetings, must stay informed about the issues before the board, and must be prepared to ask the right questions during deliberations.

The board can be sure it meets the duty of care by routinely reviewing the organization's mission, vision, and goals. The board also needs to make sure its committees have updated charters that outline the duties and responsibilities of each committee. Additionally, the board should have continuing education sessions to ensure members understand or learn how to analyze the feasibility of projects being contemplated. The board should be knowledgeable about all reasonably available information related to proposals being reviewed and act with appropriate prudence and care.

## The Duty of Loyalty

The second legal responsibility of a board is *the duty of loyalty*. The duty of loyalty requires a director to act in the best interests of the organization and its stakeholders, not of himself, a relative, or another organization with which he is affiliated. A board member should not use his position for profit, gain, or other personal advantage. The following are some specific applications of the duty of loyalty:

- **Conflict of interest.** Each director should be aware of any interest she may have that may conflict with the best interests of the organization. For example, a board member may not enter into a contract with the hospital without full disclosure and approval from the rest of the board. (See Appendix 1 for a sample conflict of interest policy and Appendix 2 for a sample conflict of interest disclosure statement.)
- **Corporate opportunity.** The duty of loyalty requires that a director not accept a business opportunity related to the business of the hospital without making that opportunity available to the hospital first. To open a business in competition with the hospital would indeed be considered bad form. Whether such an opportunity should first be offered to the hospital depends on how that opportunity relates to the hospital's existing business, how the director became aware of the opportunity, and how much interest the hospital has in the opportunity. The board should also consider how reasonable it is for the hospital to expect the director to make that opportunity available.

To meet its duty of loyalty, the board should review its conflict of interest policy and conflict of interest disclosure statement every year. Additionally, the board (or a designated committee) should review the revised Form 990 before it is filed with the IRS. The revised Form 990 helps clarify who is considered an independent director and what is considered a conflict of interest.

In summary, to meet the duty of loyalty, the board must discharge its duties unselfishly, to benefit only the organization and not the directors personally.

## The Duty of Obedience

The third legal responsibility of a board is *the duty of obedience*, which requires directors to obey all laws and support the mission and bylaws of the organization. Exceeding their delegated authority violates the trust of the organization's supporters and, in a nonprofit organization, could jeopardize its tax-exempt status. Officers and directors of healthcare organizations can be named as defendants in lawsuits filed against their organizations. And although some statutes provide a level of immunity to directors, and most organizations have directors and officers (D & O) insurance, directors should pay special attention to the limits of their authority within the organization. The board should not venture beyond those boundaries without the permission required by the hospital's operating documents.

The board helps meet its duty of obedience by not accepting proposals that are contrary to the organization's mission. The board (or designated committee) should routinely receive reports about the organization's corporate compliance program. Additionally, the board should assess community benefit performance and determine whether these activities warrant having tax-exempt status. Maintaining tax-exempt status depends on providing a certain amount of charity care each year. Board members should be aware of how the hospital is performing, especially as more state attorneys general are measuring compliance on this front. In summary, the board must ensure that the organization is obedient to its central purposes as stated in its articles of incorporation and its mission.

## COMMITTEES

Committees help the board perform its duties and meet its responsibilities. The rules regarding the type and number of committees a hospital or health system board should have are limited. However, the last thing a board should do is have too many committees, requiring members to attend more meetings than necessary. The board should appoint only those standing committees necessary to handle ongoing matters and ensure that the right members serve on them. Ad hoc committees can be formed to deal with short-term issues or a specific task, disbanding when that task is accomplished. All committees should help the process of governance and not address obvious management functions.

In addition to helping the board work efficiently, committees can play another useful role within the organization: a training ground for potential board members. Recruiting talented people to the board can be challenging, but appointing nondirector volunteers to committees is an excellent way to determine if someone would make a good board member in the future and to interest that individual in such service. However, no committee should ever be chaired by a non–board member.

In general, a healthcare organization needs the following standing committees to function effectively.

## Executive Committee

The executive committee enables a board to conduct urgent business when a regular meeting is not in session and the full board cannot readily be convened. The only caveat to having an executive committee is to not let it meet regularly. Generally speaking, if an executive committee has scheduled meetings, key decisions begin to be made solely by the executive committee, to be rubberstamped by the full board. The committee then evolves into a powerful group, leaving the rest of the board members feeling like second-class citizens.

The makeup of the executive committee should be stated in the bylaws and should include the officers of the board and other leaders, such as committee chairs. As the board's leader in residence, the CEO should be on the executive committee, except where prohibited by state statute, and should be a voting member. The CEO will obviously be excused when the committee evaluates her performance or compensation. The bylaws must clearly define the role and authority of the executive in relation to the full board.

Without such clarity, it is far too easy for the executive committee to morph into the organization's main decision-making body, with other board members losing interest and motivation or even resenting the executive committee members entirely.

> **Key Functions of the Executive Committee**
> - Providing advice to the board chair on the appointment of committees and committee chairs
> - Serving as a sounding board for the CEO
> - Helping the chair develop the governance goals and objectives for the coming year
> - Determining CEO compensation
> - Directing the CEO evaluation process

## Audit Committee

In most healthcare organizations, the audit function has historically been overseen by the finance committee or one of its subcommittees. Although the Sarbanes-Oxley Act's (Public Law 107-204, July, 2002) new regulations originally applied to publicly traded companies only, many of these requirements are now being used to evaluate nonprofit organizations, such as hospitals and health systems. In response, many organizations have established an audit committee that reports directly to the board. Almost 94 percent of nonprofit organizations reported having both an audit and a finance committee (NACD 2010b).

Recent legislative changes—including new requirements for IRS Form 990, laws applying Sarbanes-Oxley requirements to nonprofit organizations, and healthcare reform legislation that is certain to affect hospital finances—have essentially mandated that hospitals have an audit committee separate from the finance committee. The functions of the committees are so different they cannot and should not be combined.

The audit committee should consist of independent, financially literate directors, with the chair being a financial expert as defined by Sarbanes-Oxley. Although the definition of "expert" is still fuzzy, the chair should have a demonstrated understanding of auditing procedures—a professional auditor or certified public accountant is the best bet for this committee. The audit committee does not need to meet as often as the finance committee, but its functions are important to the full board.

The primary purposes of an audit committee are to foster and oversee strong financial reporting and controls and to identify and manage risk—the array of forces that may have a negative impact on the organization's financial condition. Hospitals and other healthcare organizations should consider appointing audit committees that report directly to the board and are responsible for the appointment, compensation, and oversight of the independent auditors who must report to the audit committee. Some specific functions of the audit committee include

- recommending the selection and compensation of the external auditors to the board,
- overseeing the hospital's internal audit function for the board,
- reviewing and being responsible for financial reporting and controls,
- reviewing and assessing the organization's business risk-management process,
- pre-approving any nonauditing functions proposed by the external auditors,
- reviewing and approving the code of ethical financial conduct,
- defining significant conflicts of interest and related-party transactions, and
- performing both the external and internal audit functions.


## Finance Committee

The finance committee helps the board maintain and improve the financial integrity of the organization. Specific functions of the finance committee include

- drafting finance policies for board review and adoption;
- developing key financial ratios to be used by the committee and specific ratios for the board;

- reviewing the draft budget, including revenues, expenses, and capital expenditures for the coming year, and recommending its adoption to the board; and
- completing a regular review of all board policies and decisions regarding finances.

## Governance Committee

The governance committee is charged with oversight of the board's composition, organization, work processes, and effectiveness. This committee oversees the evaluation of individual board members and the board as a whole. In addition, the governance committee evaluates itself every year. Individual board member assessments are a delicate matter requiring the utmost levels of tact, candor, and confidentiality. Like full-board evaluations, the focus of individual director evaluations should be on performance and not on personality. See appendixes 3 and 4 for a sample individual board member performance appraisal. Specific functions of the governance committee include

- clarifying the duties and responsibilities of the board and its members,
- evaluating board structure and composition,
- nominating members to the board,
- monitoring policies and practices of the board,
- planning the annual board retreat,
- designing the new-member orientation process,
- directing the board's continuing education and development activities,
- completing the board's self-assessment process,
- analyzing the results of the self-assessment process, and
- regularly reviewing all board policies and decisions regarding governance performance.

## Planning Committee

The planning committee, sometimes called the strategic planning committee, helps the board formulate policies; develop goals and objectives; and determine the organization's overall, big-picture strategic direction. Specific duties of the planning committee include

- developing and recommending the strategic plan for the organization;
- developing mechanisms to monitor that plan and recommend needed updates, additions, or amendments;

- occasionally completing an analysis of key stakeholders, which will include their interests and expectations, as well as a physician staffing plan; and
- reviewing proposals submitted by management for board recommendations.

## Quality and Community Health Committee

This committee's work assures the board that the organization is providing quality care and addressing the health of the community. At one time, this committee might have only involved itself in what went on inside the hospital's walls. However, in today's competitive environment, healthcare organizations should broaden their scope of involvement into the entire community; therefore, this committee must broaden its own scope accordingly. Additionally, part of healthcare reform legislation requires hospitals to complete regular community health needs-assessment studies.

With an expanded scope, the quality and community health committee must have equal footing with the audit and finance committees. When boards make it clear the quality and community health committee is vital, they send a message to the administration, the medical staff, and others that quality matters and must be taken seriously. Specific duties of the quality and community health committee include

- ensuring systems for measuring quality care in the hospital or health system are established, meaningful, and regularly reviewed;
- drafting policies regarding all aspects of quality for review and adoption by the board;
- identifying the community's health status and needs and recommending actions the hospital could take to improve;
- identifying potential collaborations with other community health providers to enhance community health status; and
- diligently reviewing medical staff recommendations regarding appointment, reappointment, and privilege delineation of physicians.

## RESPONSIBILITIES OF INDIVIDUAL BOARD MEMBERS

Board members frequently accept their roles with enthusiasm, tempered with hesitance about being the new kid on the block. Those who have been around a while can either become comfortable with their roles or become jaded and lax. Individual board members are responsible for fulfilling the duty of care, the duty of loyalty, and the duty of obedience. A sample job description is provided on page 19.

Ideally, individual board members will continually contribute to the advancement of the organization because they do the following:

- **Understand the organization.** Board members need to understand and believe in the organization's mission, vision, goals, objectives, and bylaws. Agreement with the mission is particularly important as it drives all decisions. If board members have the mission of the organization clearly in mind, most decisions will be easy to make.

- **Develop a broad knowledge of the healthcare industry.** Board members are not necessarily expected to be experts, but they need to develop a broad knowledge of the healthcare industry and trends. The CEO can be helpful in providing educational materials for this purpose. Members should also attend educational programs, read a few healthcare journals, and stay abreast of industry news. This is particularly important with the passage of the healthcare reform bill.

- **Acquire a working knowledge of committee subject matter.** Individual board members should acquire a fundamental knowledge about the functional areas related to their committee assignments. For example, a board member on the finance committee should seek out articles and materials related to finance committees of healthcare organizations. Again, the CEO can be helpful in giving board members materials to read and suggesting seminars to attend.

- **Prepare.** Before meetings, board members should read all provided materials so that they can deliberate intelligently during the meeting. Sometimes board members (particularly new ones) hesitate to ask questions or request information because they are intimidated by hospital jargon and medical terminology. A board member should never hesitate to ask questions or to indicate something he does not understand. Board members should remember that serving on a hospital board is not their usual day job, and they are not expected to know what management, physicians, or more seasoned board members know about hospital operations. That knowledge will come with experience and preparation.

- **Regularly attend meetings—on time.** Board members are expected to attend all board and committee meetings, arrive on time, and execute their assignments on time. In today's healthcare environment, a board cannot afford to have "letterhead" directors—people whose names appear on the organization's stationery but who do not attend meetings. These ornamental directors are essentially useless to the organization.

- **Make a positive contribution.** A board member must make a positive contribution to board discussions, always keeping in mind the best interests of the organization. This allows the board to reach sound conclusions and speak with one voice; there should be no minority reports. Even if a vote was as close as 5 to 4, it is inappropriate for an individual board member to indicate to someone outside of the board that a decision was a bad one and she voted against it. The board must be clear that this is not acceptable behavior and must act to remove a repeat offender from the board to preserve its effectiveness, teamwork, and credibility in the community. In county and district hospitals where members come from varied sources, this enforcement can be difficult to accomplish, but the offending member must at least be counseled away from such destructive behavior.

- **Do not dominate meetings.** Board members who dominate discussions, ignore the agenda, or digress to their own interests create problems for the board and for the CEO. An effective board chair will not allow this to happen, and other board members can also help keep the meeting on track. Such behavior should be considered during the offending member's evaluation.

- **Avoid rumors and gossip.** Board members should ask the CEO or the board president about any rumors, gossip, or criticism of the hospital they encounter before drawing conclusions. This will allow the board and the CEO to work in tandem to handle incorrect information in an appropriate fashion.

- **Avoid conflict of interest.** In today's turbulent environment, board members cannot have or give even the appearance of having a conflict of interest.

   As an example, consider a hospital board in a town with five banks. Bill is a board member and also president of the bank where the hospital deposits its money. The finance committee has recommended the hospital look at other banks to find a more competitive interest rate. The board chair says, "Bill, we're going to look at moving the hospital's money from your bank to another bank in town, so you better step out of the room and abstain from this discussion and vote because of your possible conflict of interest." Bill steps out of the room and after its discussion, the board decides to switch banks. The chair calls Bill back and says, "Well, Bill, we decided to move the hospital's money to XYZ bank. I hope you don't have a problem with that decision." What would be the likelihood of Bill being a cooperative, team-playing board member during the next few years? In another scenario, the rest of the board members could decide not to move the hospital's money out of loyalty to Bill rather than loyalty to the best interest of the hospital. This decision would also be inappropriate.

   The best solution then is to avoid placing an individual on the board who could have, or could appear to have, a conflict of interest in the first place. Again, because district or county hospital board members must be elected or appointed, those hospitals have a particular difficulty in accomplishing this and must be extremely sensitive in this area. (Appendix 1 provides a sample conflict of interest policy, and Appendix 2 provides a sample conflict of interest disclosure statement.)

- **Avoid interfering in hospital operations.** This topic is a pitfall for many board members. The board needs to look at the strategic direction of the organization from 30,000 feet, where its members can see where the organization is going without getting involved in the details of getting there. If board members are functioning at the 5,000-feet level, they have crossed the line from governance to management. Sometimes board members get involved in operations because the CEO has given them management information instead of governance information. For example, governance information might include strategic planning specifics, information about possible mergers or major service changes, the overall financial picture, or financial and quality dashboard indicators. Management information would include such details as the color or design of a remodeled lobby, reviewing the points in a managed care contract, or the financial records of individual department spending. If the board receives governance information, it might just govern; but it will certainly try to manage if it receives detailed management information.

- **Maintain hospital confidentiality.** Board members who share confidential information with outside parties present a real problem for the hospital and for the CEO. Certain board deliberations are most appropriately left in the boardroom, with publicity properly directed to final board action and not the discussions that led to that action. Board members should remember to check with the board chair or the CEO if they have questions about how much and what type of information can be shared. It is the board's duty to keep confidential information inside the boardroom.

- **Be a partner to the CEO.** Even though the board is responsible for hiring and evaluating the CEO, directors should act like partners and advisers to the CEO rather than supervisors. The organization has a much better chance of success if the board and the CEO are functioning as a team; there will also be a greater satisfaction level for both and a greater benefit to the organization if this teamwork exists. Board members must be honest and candid with the CEO. Discussing key issues behind the CEO's back leads to an unhealthy relationship.

- **Serve as a mentor/consultant.** Any individual board member should be available to serve as a consultant or sounding board to the CEO and others in the organization. Seasoned board members can also be helpful to new members as they learn their role in the organization and on the board.

- **Be alert for new opportunities.** As hospitals are increasingly expected to assume some responsibility for their community's health, board members are in key positions to identify areas of need the hospital might fill. Of course, by virtue of their occupations and positions, some board members have better opportunities for this than others, but all should be alert to this responsibility.
- **Interpret the hospital to the community.** The individual board member should be a representative of the hospital, interpreting it and its functions to the community. Though they must always remember the need to keep certain information confidential, and the need for the board to speak with one voice, board members can be extremely influential in gathering support for the hospital and its programs.

As a side note, many hospitals lose or ignore their retired board members, but these individuals can also be helpful if they continue their positive relationship with the organization. With a little effort on the hospital's part, retired board members can stay informed and appropriately involved, and they can do wonders for the hospital in the community.

## RESPONSIBILITIES OF THE BOARD CHAIR

Eight basic responsibilities of a board chair are described below, and a sample job description for a board chair is provided at the end of this chapter. Each chair brings unique strengths and weaknesses to the role but should ensure these responsibilities are carried out. The board chair

1. **Serves as a counselor to the CEO.** The chair counsels the CEO on governance matters and board–CEO relations. There is possibly no more important function the chair fulfills. The chair and the CEO must work together as a team, with the chair serving as a sounding board and marshaling board support for the CEO. The chair can also help the CEO clarify her goals and objectives for the coming year.
2. **Presides over all meetings of the board and executive committee.** The board chair should be able to run focused, creative, effective, and efficient board meetings. A chair who does not know how to preside over a meeting wastes everyone's time and energy. If the chair does not possess these skills, he should learn them—fast.
3. **Designates board committees.** With the advice and consent of the executive committee, the chair designates board committees and committee chairs. The

executive committee provides a good check for the chair's selections. Additionally, the chair should mentor and advise the committee chairs.

4. **Serves as an ex officio member of all committees.** The chair is not necessarily expected to attend all board committee meetings, but she should be kept up to date on committee activities.

5. **Serves as the board's representative.** The chair represents the board to the community at large and to key stakeholder groups.

6. **Specifies annual objectives, work plans, and meeting agendas.** With assistance provided by the executive committee and the CEO, the chair develops annual objectives for the board, determining its priorities in relation to its own functions. The chair will develop the board's work plan and formulate agendas (with the CEO) for all board meetings.

7. **Serves as a mentor.** The chair serves as a role model and mentor for future chairs and other board members. Working through others (particularly the CEO), the chair is responsible for recruitment, orientation, and development of all board members, including the evaluation of board members (which may actively involve the governance committee).

8. **Assumes other responsibilities and tasks as directed by the board.** The chair may perform other functions as requested by the board. But it is the chair's responsibility to ensure the board stays focused on those things that fit the mission, vision, and goals of the organization and that it follows established policy and procedure to keep people on task. No one has more influence on the board's success, so it is important for the board and the chair to be in sync. The board does not want a personality-driven chair who may steer the organization in the wrong strategic direction. To ensure consistency from one board chair to the next, the chair must not lead the board off into an area of personal interest. The chair functions as an instrument of the board, not the other way around.

## JOB DESCRIPTIONS

A common cause of ineffective governance is confusion among board members about their roles and responsibilities. In addition, there is often confusion about a hospital board's role in relation to a health system board's role and the authority limit levels of each (see page 21). Having job descriptions for officers and directors may be one of the most important ways to improve a board's performance.

The most fundamental characteristic of excellent governance is that all board members have a shared understanding of their jobs. Boards are not all alike, and they have a different mix of skills and personalities. Each board should answer for itself a basic question: What is the job of board members of *this* hospital? Board member job descriptions can serve several important purposes, such as

- **Orientation.** A good job description explains the roles and responsibilities of the new board member, which helps the new board member to become oriented more quickly.
- **Recruitment.** Job descriptions help the governance committee concentrate on finding new board members with the set of skills the board needs at that time. Potential new board members will know exactly what will be expected of them.
- **Self-assessment.** Good job descriptions can help the governance committee develop an effective self-assessment program for the board or individual members.
- **Managing multiple boards.** Many hospitals are part of health systems that have more than one board. Uncertainty about when each board has the authority to act can be reduced with good job descriptions. Also, clear delineation of each board's roles and responsibilities will reduce the conflict among multiple boards.
- **Separating governance and management.** Clear job descriptions (for the board and CEO) can explain the differences between governance and management responsibilities. Confusion about governance functions and management functions can lead to friction between the board and staff.

Sample basic job descriptions for a board chair, board vice chair, and an individual board member of a hospital or health system are provided. However, each organization will undoubtedly wish to customize its own documents.

## SAMPLE JOB DESCRIPTION: CHAIR OF THE BOARD

Function: The chair, in addition to serving as a member of the board and executive committee, represents the highest level of the board and works cooperatively with the organization's CEO. The chair is responsible for ensuring the integrity and effectiveness of the board's governance role and processes.

The chair of the board presides at all meetings of the board of directors and the executive committee; oversees implementation of corporate (if applicable) and local policies; and manages the actions and directions of the board in accordance with its bylaws, mission, vision, and goals.

*(continued)*

The chair represents the board within the hospital and the hospital in the community.

**Responsibilities**

- Serves as counselor/adviser to the CEO on matters of governance and board relations
- Directs the board and facilitates meetings of the board and executive committee
- Calls special meetings of the board when necessary
- Designates board committee memberships and chairs of board committees, with the advice and consent of the executive committee
- Serves as ex-officio member of all board committees—standing and ad hoc
- With the CEO and executive committee, formulates annual objectives for the board, determines the board's priorities, and creates a work plan for the year
- With the CEO, formulates board meeting agendas
- Sets an example for and mentors other board members and committee chairs
- Ensures that board members focus discussions on the goals of the organization
- Delegates or executes the policies established by the board
- Working with the executive committee, monitors the performance of the CEO, including annual performance and salary reviews
- Working with the governance committee, completes a regular evaluation of individual board members and the board as a whole
- Works closely with the vice chair to develop and implement officer transition plans
- Aids in the recruitment and orientation of new board members
- If the hospital board is part of a health system that has other boards, including a parent board, is responsible for knowing specifically what duties and authority have been delegated to his board
- Assumes other responsibilities and tasks as directed by the board

## SAMPLE JOB DESCRIPTION: VICE CHAIR OF THE BOARD

Function: The vice chair of the board, in addition to serving as a member of the board and executive committee, fulfills the duties of the chair in the event of her absence or disability and performs other duties as may be assigned by the board or the chair.

**Responsibilities**

- Performs the duties of the chair in her absence
- Serves on the executive committee
- May chair at least one major committee

- Helps the chair monitor the implementation of board-established policies
- With the other officers, monitors the performance of the CEO
- With the other officers and the governance committee, conducts regular performance evaluations of individual board members and the board as a whole
- Works closely with the chair to develop and implement officer transition plans

## SAMPLE JOB DESCRIPTION: BOARD MEMBER

Function: A board member participates in the governance of the hospital or health system, including the establishment and implementation of board policies, in accordance with its bylaws, mission, vision, and goals.

**Responsibilities**
- Prepares for and attends all annual, regular, and special board meetings; reads all agenda materials in advance of such meetings
- Participates in the affairs of the board in accordance with the organization's mission, vision, and goals
- Fulfills the duty of care, the duty of loyalty, and the duty of obedience
- Understands and upholds the organization's code of ethics; avoids potential personal and professional conflicts of interest
- Is not accountable to any special group or interest, and acts and makes decisions that are in the best interest of the hospital as a whole
- Establishes corporate policy
- Employs the organization's top management
- Helps establish evaluation criteria for the CEO; monitors and applies the criteria to stimulate, support, reward, and, when necessary or desirable, change top management
- Avoids interfering in hospital operations (understands the difference between governance and management)
- Reviews results achieved by management in keeping with the hospital's mission and goals
- Develops and recommends strategic directions and financial plans for the hospital
- Approves annual budgets
- Keeps all board deliberations confidential
- Participates in board orientation and continuing education
- Participates in the board self-appraisals

*(continued)*

- Serves on board committees and gains knowledge about their functions
- May chair a board committee
- Elects officers at annual board meetings
- Represents the hospital to the community
- Is knowledgeable about the stakeholders to whom the hospital is accountable
- Participates in fundraising activities
- If the hospital is part of a health system, is responsible for understanding the board's limits of authority

## ONLINE RESOURCES FOR BOARD GOVERNANCE INFORMATION

For the board member who has some time to learn about the healthcare industry, how boards should function, and best practices of governance, the following websites are worth reviewing:

1. **BoardSource (www.boardsource.org).** BoardSource is a resource for practical information, tools and best practices, training, and leadership development for board members of nonprofit organizations worldwide. Through its educational programs and services, BoardSource works to help organizations fulfill their missions by building strong and effective nonprofit boards.
2. **Center for Healthcare Governance (www.americangovernance.com).** Backed by the knowledge and resources of the American Hospital Association, the Center for Healthcare Governance provides state-of-the-art education, research, publications, services, tools, and other governance resources to help boards achieve and maintain consistency and excellence throughout their governance program.
3. **Corporate Directors Forum (www.directorsforum.com).** The Corporate Directors Forum is dedicated to promoting high standards of professionalism in corporate board directorship. It forges alliances among leadership in industry, academia, and government to generate corporate stakeholder values, while fostering high standards of ethics, diversity, and social responsibility. It also provides board-focused peer networking, best practices directorship education, governance advocacy leadership, director mentoring, and board recruitment resources.
4. **The Corporate Library (www.thecorporatelibrary.com).** The Corporate Library is intended to serve as a central repository for research, study, and criti-

cal thinking about the nature of the modern corporation, with a special focus on governance and the relationship between management and the board of directors. Most general content on the site is open to visitors at no cost; however, advanced research relating to specific companies and certain other advanced features are restricted to subscribers only.

5. **The Governance Institute (www.governanceinstitute.com).** The Governance Institute provides an education and development subscription service designed exclusively for health system and hospital boards. Benefits include on-demand research services, access to the institute's governance information clearinghouse, copies of research reports and white papers, copies of the bimonthly Board Room Press for all directors, and educational videos on key healthcare issues.

6. **National Association of Corporate Directors (www.nacdonline.org).** Founded in 1977, the National Association of Corporate Directors (NACD) is an educational, publishing, and consulting organization focused on board leadership. In addition, it is a membership association for boards, directors, director-candidates, and board advisors. NACD promotes professional board standards, creates forums for peer interaction, enhances director effectiveness, asserts the policy interests of directors, conducts research, and educates boards and directors concerning traditional and cutting-edge issues.

## References

American College of Healthcare Executives (ACHE). 2010. "Top Issues Confronting Hospitals: 2009." *Healthcare Executive* 25 (2): 98.

Kaiser, L. 2011. Personal Communication.

Kazemek, E. A. 2002. "Count to Ten: Board and CEO Frustrations." *Trustee* 55 (9): 26–27.

National Association of Corporate Directors (NACD). 2010a. "2009–2010 NACD Public Company Governance Survey." Washington, DC: National Association of Corporate Directors.

———. 2010b. 2009 NACD Nonprofit Governance Survey. Washington, DC: National Association of Corporate Directors.

# CHAPTER TWO

# How to Operate Your Board

All hospital trustees know being a board member today is much more difficult than it was even five years ago. With healthcare reform and other changes in the industry, hospitals and health systems must have boards that function smoothly and comprise the best talent available.

## OPTIMUM BOARD SIZE

Does the size of your board help or hinder its work? Many boards face this question in this age of increased pressure on healthcare organizations. While many boards can determine their own size, the boards of county, district, or city hospitals essentially have no say in the matter, as that has been determined by their creating authorities.

Many nonprofit boards tend to be larger than they should be, having grown too quickly in their formative years. Historically, hospitals wanted to retain support from as many stakeholder groups as possible; a seat on the board provided concrete evidence of the esteem the hospital had for the stakeholder group. Likewise, many hospitals wanted to have as many potential donors on the board as possible; representation from major community corporations brought those companies into the hospital's family. Some hospitals also wanted geographic representation, particularly if they provided care in a large service area in a county or to several counties.

Today, however, the board must look critically at membership to find what is needed for the good of the organization, not as a reward or incentive to contribute.

Many studies have found the most effective board size is 9 to 17 members; health system boards average 16 to 17 members, while nonprofit hospital boards average 13 to 14 members (Prybil 2008).

As a comparison, when NACD (2010a) completed a study on the optimum size of boards for public companies, almost 60 percent of the respondents said a board should range from 8 to 11 members; the average size is 9.1, a small increase over the past three years. One reason for the increase may be that boards are recruiting more directors to broaden the board's available skill sets.

When NACD (2010b) completed its survey of nonprofit corporations, almost 74 percent of directors thought having 11 to 17 members was "just right." Almost 50 percent thought that 18 members was too many for a board. Interestingly, however, the average size of the nonprofit boards surveyed by NACD was 19.8.

Although each board will need to determine its own magic number, as a general starting point, boards of fewer than nine are usually too small and boards of more than 18 are too large. With fewer than nine members, it becomes easy for a few loud individuals to exercise more influence than might be healthy. With more than 18, it can be difficult to reach a consensus, keep all board members up to date, and make timely decisions in a turbulent environment. There are always exceptions. For example, one district hospital board in Northern California has a five-member board, and each member serves on several committees, which seems to work for that hospital. When evaluating their board's size, members should consider:

- What work needs to be done
- What kind of expertise and skills would be useful
- How current members cope with the required workload
- How the current size of the board meets the organization's needs.

Any changes in size can then be linked to the needs of the hospital rather than to the personalities of individual directors. In general, hospital and health system boards in the 10- to 17-seat range seem to reach decisions and function more efficiently than do larger or smaller boards.

## FREQUENCY OF BOARD MEETINGS

Traditionally, healthcare boards met monthly. More recently, an increasing number of boards have begun moving to meeting every other month or quarterly. Recent surveys by NACD (2010a; 2010b) show that boards of publicly traded corporations and nonprofits meet about six times per year. Studies now show that more than 50 percent of hospitals and health systems are meeting fewer than nine times per year, and half of those are meeting six times per year or less (Prybil 2008; Alexander 1990). Effective boards are meeting less often and still achieving results:

- **Improved recruitment.** Finding and recruiting good, experienced board members can be difficult. If potential board members perceive that your board is efficient and effective and uses time prudently, they are more likely to join you. If your board seems to meet whether it needs to or not or spends time on trivial or management matters instead of governance, the response will likely be less positive.
- **More efficient use of time and information.** A board that meets quarterly instead of monthly is forced to use time efficiently, making it essential for the organization's staff to provide governance information instead of management information. Many board members will not say anything about receiving unnecessary information; they just won't read it. Eventually, they may read nothing at all in advance of the meeting, affecting the board's efficiency and effectiveness. The board should insist on a biannual review of all the reports it receives so that members can indicate which they find inappropriate and can focus solely on governance information. Members will then be more inclined to read their materials, assured that what they receive is indeed important to their purpose.
- **More effective delegation to committees.** Much of a board's work is done in committees. Effective boards make sure the right people lead and serve on the committees. If the committees are structured and staffed with careful thought, the board is less likely to duplicate the committee's work, and therefore the board can meet less frequently. Choosing the committee chairs is one of the most important jobs of the board chair.

If a board finds it difficult to meet quarterly, it might move to meeting six times per year to start. True to human nature, boards tend to fill the amount of time allotted for a meeting. By reducing that time, members usually become aware of the need for more efficient meetings and look for ways to make this happen.

## INFORMATION NEEDED FOR BOARD MEETINGS

Boards must receive governance information rather than management information. All materials for discussion at a meeting should be sent to board members at least a week before any meeting. What should these different materials include?

**Board Meeting Materials**

- **Minutes of the previous meeting.** The board should receive minutes from the previous meeting to give members a chance to refresh their memories about the discussions and the actions taken. Minutes should be brief but thorough and should reflect action taken without a verbatim account of the discussion.
- **Agenda for the coming meeting.** The CEO should spend enough time with the board chair to develop a thoughtful and meaningful agenda addressing the key issues and reports in a logical sequence.
- **Complete financial statements.** The board must receive complete financial statements at each meeting, along with dashboard financial indicators—the specific items the finance committee and board have agreed are particularly meaningful and that the board wishes to see in more detail at each meeting.

**Responsibilities**

- **A quality measurement report.** The board should always receive a meaningful, concise quality measurement report from a physician or nurse. The report should contain quality indicators developed by the quality and community health committee and agreed to by the board, just as are the financial indicators developed by the finance committee.
- **Other reports and resource materials.** In addition to a progress report from the CEO and reports from its other board committees, the board should periodically receive materials regarding trends in healthcare. These resources should be educational and should help the board think strategically as it considers future options for the organization.

Many boards receive entirely too much information, which members frequently do not bother to read. One giveaway is the member who arrives at a meeting with an obviously unopened packet of materials and who does not or cannot contribute to the discussion. Another is the report nobody seems to know much about and that never gets discussed. When queried about why it received such a report, one board member in Wyoming replied, "Bill insisted we get it, and it just keeps coming." When asked why Bill wasn't at that particular meeting so he could be asked about it, the answer was, "Oh, Bill died four years ago."

To address these problems, at least every two years the full board should review and evaluate the type of information it is receiving. Changes can then be made based on members' needs and suggestions.

## EXECUTIVE SESSIONS

Between the Sarbanes-Oxley law, the Securities and Exchange Commission (SEC), and rules for both stock markets (NASDAQ and the New York Stock Exchange), almost all boards of public corporations are required to conduct regular executive sessions of their independent directors. The SEC maintains that regularly scheduled executive sessions encourage and enhance communication among independent directors. The laws mandate that executive sessions will occur at least twice a year and perhaps more frequently, in conjunction with regularly scheduled board meetings. Board members of public corporations who are also board members of hospitals see the value of regular executive sessions and appear to support this board practice as hospital board members.

Executive sessions—in which the board directors meet without the CEO and hospital staff—can be a sensitive subject between boards and CEOs. However, boards who conduct regular executive sessions know this may allow the board to talk more thoroughly about a wider range of issues than just CEO compensation and evaluation. Executive sessions also allow a board to explore issues that may not be clearly understood by some board members but about which they are hesitant to ask in an open public meeting.

If an executive session is part of board policy, it can remove the natural anxiety the CEO or other staff members might feel about not being included. The board, including the CEO, should have an open discussion on executive session policy and its pros and cons. Alternatively, the board's governance committee could develop an executive session policy.

The American Hospital Association's Health Research and Educational Trust and its Center for Healthcare Governance conducted a survey regarding executive sessions, with 350 hospital CEOs responding (Alexander 1990). Overall, nearly 90 percent of the boards had held at least one executive session in the past two years, but most averaged between one and eight such sessions per year. CEOs from smaller hospitals were more likely than CEOs from larger hospitals or health systems to attend the whole executive session.

## SELECTING A BOARD CHAIR

Next to selecting a CEO, the most important thing a board can do is elect the right person to be board chair. A good chair does not necessarily guarantee high levels of board effectiveness, but a bad one guarantees ineffective performance.

When making this determination, all board members must remember: The chair does not control the board; the board controls the chair. If the board allows the chair to control the direction and activities of the board, then every time a new chair is selected, the organization may head off in a different direction, losing stability and continuity.

Although all board members should serve with no term limits, they should definitely limit the number of years or terms an individual may serve as chair. Generally, a board chair should not serve more than four to six years; the bylaws need to clearly address the matter as well as whether or not there will be a chair-elect in the mix. The individual who has been serving as chair may remain on the board following her term, provided she is nominated again for a board seat and wishes to continue serving as a board member.

Being a board chair today requires energy and time; serving much longer than four to six years will burn many chairs out, and they will no longer be able to give their best to the position. As Orlikoff and Totten (2008) point out, chairs without term limits pose certain risks for the board, such as prolonged ineffective leadership due to the position becoming personality-driven rather than mission-driven. Boards usually hesitate to vote an incumbent chair out of office, and other members may become frustrated and leave if they see no possibility of leadership change on the horizon. In addition, effective board chair succession planning usually does not occur without term limits clearly establishing the parameters of the office. Do not put your chair in a position to burn out or put your board in the position of wishing the chair was not in the position any longer.

In addition to having term limits for the chair, the board may want to consider adopting the chair-elect model. The board would then have a system for determining who the next chair will be, a year before the present chair finishes his final term. That gives the chair-elect a year to watch and learn from the serving board chair, a year for the board to get used to whom the next chair will be, and time for a smooth transition from one leader to the next.

The board chair should periodically be evaluated by the board, in the same way individual board members are evaluated. Regularly assessing board chair performance can make a good chair even better. A thorough board chair evaluation process involves

- a written job description,
- a clearly defined process, and
- a time frame for the evaluation process to occur.

The board should consider the following questions when electing a board chair (or chair-elect):

1. Does this individual have the time and energy to devote to the position?
2. Will this individual be effective in providing a confidential sounding board for the CEO?
3. Does this individual demonstrate a good understanding of the organization and its long-term goals (e.g., has this person had a long enough tenure on the board)?
4. Does this individual understand the board's role as policymaker?
5. Does this individual know the difference between governance and management?
6. Does this individual come to meetings prepared?
7. Does this individual make valuable contributions? Does she raise pertinent questions and provide valuable insights?
8. Is this individual respected by her board colleagues?
9. Is this individual a good listener who considers other perspectives before making decisions?
10. Does this individual understand the balance between discussing an issue fully and reaching decisions in a timely fashion?

Given the variables in human nature, some people who are great board members may be ineffective board chairs. There are those who are not comfortable in that kind of leadership position but who otherwise make invaluable contributions to the board's work. A smart board will not place someone in the role of chair if he does not wish to sit there.


## TERM LIMITS

(Adapted from *Trustee*, Vol. 54, No. 2, by permission, February 2001. Copyright 2001, by Health Forum, Inc.)

Serving as a board member is a challenge. Nearly all hospitals operate in competitive environments where reimbursement is constantly changing and where physicians fight to maintain their incomes, often in direct competition with the hospital. Many hospitals functioning in this environment have term limits for board members. Many governance experts recommend term limits to ensure turnover of board members. However, it is becoming more apparent that board term limits must be reexamined.

Many hospitals lose some of their best board members because of term limits. In a survey of directors of publicly traded companies (NACD 2010a), less than 10 percent had term limits and almost 68 percent completed annual evaluations of individual board members. In NACD's survey of directors of nonprofit corporations (2010b), less than one-third had term limits and almost 85 percent completed annual evaluations of individual board members, up from about 40 percent a year earlier. It is estimated that about half of hospital and health system boards do not have term limits (Prybil 2008).

## Primary Disadvantage of Term Limits

Hospitals are complex organizations and are often the largest employer in a community. Service from knowledgeable and talented board members is required. However, in today's healthcare environment, recruiting talented board members is becoming more difficult. And once recruited, no matter how talented they are, board members often need two to four years of education to understand the healthcare industry and hospitals in particular. To lose such knowledgeable and experienced board members because of arbitrary term limits is counterproductive.

## Another Approach

Rather than losing members to term limits, it makes more sense to complete a periodic performance appraisal of each board member and to let go of board members who score badly.

Parkview Medical Center in Pueblo, Colorado, dealt with the issue of term limits directly. The hospital board had term limits for several years and found it was losing knowledgeable, experienced, and dedicated board members as a result. More than ten years ago, the board voted to change the bylaws to eliminate term limits. The board now conducts an annual evaluation of board members and has been satisfied with this process and the performance of its individual board members.

Central Maine Medical Center in Lewiston, Maine, also voted to eliminate term limits. The results have been positive, and the board now has a group of stable, talented, and committed board members.

## Annual Selection

Inova Health System, a five-hospital system in Northern Virginia, appointed a governance committee to research options for board member selection. After reviewing the usual methods of selecting board members, the board decided to elect board members annually, and to elect the chair for one five-year term. "The board felt this method was better than having term limits, and would keep board members focused on how they were performing on a more regular basis," says Knox Singleton, president and CEO. "This method of selecting board members has worked well for us and has helped members concentrate on their governance role and effective leadership for a large organization" (Biggs 2001).

The Washington, DC–based Health Care Advisory Board (1996) completed a study on appointing board members and recommended annual election of trustees. This enables the governance committee to determine whether to renew individual trusteeships for another year. The roles of the board chair and the governance committee become extremely important in such a system, and these individuals need to make objective and sometimes difficult decisions. Performance appraisals can help.

## Performance Appraisals

To accomplish annual selection as smoothly and objectively as possible, a formal evaluation process should be in place; ideally, the size of the board will be such that the evaluation process does not become onerous and all-consuming. This process will provide an opportunity to craft individual roles for each trustee, giving her a clear sense of the purpose and importance of her role. Annual completion of the process will give the board an opportunity to provide feedback to trustees on how they are perceived and how they can provide maximum benefit to the hospital. The process also paves the way for the board and a board member to part amicably when the member lacks certain skills or commitment. In fact, evaluation is the best way to rotate directors, and it is most effective when approached with a positive mind-set. The purpose of evaluation is not to root out "bad" or "underperforming" directors. Rather, it is to see if the board membership serves the strategic needs of the hospital. Making evaluation and rotation a regular occurrence lessens the stigma of director turnover. (Appendixes 3 and 4 provide sample evaluation forms).

The annual performance appraisal should be brief and should be completed and reviewed with the director by the board chair or the governance committee chair. If a chair-elect model is used, the chair may wish to have that individual assist with performance appraisals.

There can be as few as five to ten questions, each of which is assigned points to measure satisfactory performance. Questions can relate to the director's

- attendance,
- meeting preparation,
- understanding of role,

- willingness to take appropriate risks,
- support of board decisions,
- knowledge of the healthcare industry,
- understanding results of board decisions,
- dependability,
- ability to work with others, and
- willingness to compromise.

Performance appraisals allow the governance committee to monitor board composition over time, identify less effective trustees, and coach others to better performance.

The individual performance appraisal does not take the place of a periodic board self-assessment survey. The survey should contain questions about board performance and board perceptions. That survey is usually completed by board members and tabulated by an outside consultant, and it is a major discussion item at a board retreat. (See the "Board Self-Assessment Process and Sample Assessment Tool" later in this chapter and Exhibit 2.2 for a sample survey.)

## Chair of the Board

Although all board members should serve with no term limits, there should definitely be a limit on the number of years or terms an individual may fill the office of chair. Generally, a board chair should not serve more than four to six years as chair; the bylaws need to clearly address the matter as well as whether or not there will be a chair-elect in the mix. The individual who has been serving as chair may, however, remain on the board, provided she is nominated again for a board seat and wishes to continue serving as a board member.

Although eliminating term limits for board members makes sense, there are reasons to limit the term of the board chair to a fixed amount of time in office. According to Dr. Lee Seidel, professor of health administration at the University of Colorado (Biggs 2001):

> The board chair should change every two to four years. The learning curve is too much to [overcome] in less than two years. The chair-elect model ... forces the board to focus on who should be the next chair and provides that person with at least a year to closely observe the role and responsibilities of the chair. A person may be a very good board member, but would not make a good chairperson, which the board needs to keep in mind.

The board chair needs to have a high energy level. In today's challenging healthcare environment, most individuals have difficulty maintaining that level after four to six years as chair. Some governance observers have concluded the chair should change after a reasonable period, before he loses interest or burns out (Biggs 2001).

## AGE LIMITS

Is there a time when someone can no longer make a positive contribution to a board's work? Certainly. But that time does not arrive at some arbitrarily established age. Just as with term limits, if an effective performance appraisal process is in place and the governance committee evaluates each board member on a regular basis, age limits are not necessary. Extensive reviews of the scientific literature on aging, physical and mental abilities, and job performance lead to the conclusion that chronological age is not a good predictor of abilities or performance. McEvoy and Cascio (1989) reviewed 96 research studies spanning a 22-year period to examine the effect of age on performance; they found performance did not decrease as age increased, as is typically believed.

One 35-year study of intellectual development reported that age-related changes in cognitive functions occur slowly. For most people, declines in intellectual abilities are of a small magnitude until they reach their mid-70s (Schaie 1996). Older individuals may actually have higher motivation and job satisfaction than the young. Researchers who examined 185 studies found internal work motivation, overall job satisfaction, and job involvement were positively associated with age (Rhodes 1983).

Many of the declines formerly attributed to aging should be attributed to injury, illness, or lifestyle variables. Therefore, age averages are not good indicators of individual ability levels, and the average ability of a 60- or 70-year-old is not a useful basis for estimating individual capabilities and limitations. Generally speaking, therefore, boards should not conclude that ability declines are so uniform, common, or dramatic as to warrant putting age limits on individual board members.

According to surveys completed by NACD (2010a; 2010b), about 50 percent of publicly traded and nonprofit corporations have age limits. However, the boards having age limits are setting a more advanced age as their cap. In the 1990s, most set the age limit between 65 and 70. That number is increasing steadily and now averages about 72, with 75 or even 80 set as the limit on many boards.

From another perspective, it can be useful to have a few board members who have been around long enough to provide a "corporate memory" for the board. Despite the cliché, boards do need to learn from the past to avoid making mistakes. Understanding what has gone before can indeed help boards make better decisions; older, long-term members can be a bridge to that understanding.

Experience is also a great teacher, and board members, like all of us, learn from personal experiences. Sometimes it takes considerable time to accumulate enough experience to be able to view the healthcare organization and its community as a total system and to make the right connections. Experienced individuals, in many instances, see problems and opportunities as a whole within a complete context, which then allows them to also see obvious solutions to many problems.

Dysfunctional board members can come in all shapes, sizes, and ages. Excellent board members are excellent because they come to meetings on time, read the distributed material before the meeting, act as team players, and support board decisions. Age is not the determining factor for success on a board; other attributes clearly seem to be the important components, and these will show up when the individual is evaluated. As a delightful example, one midwestern board member is at least 86 years old, has been on his board for more than 53 years, and is generally viewed as the best overall member of that board. A large number of boards and governance committees today use evaluation, rather than retirement policies, term limits or age limits, as the way to rotate directors.

## PAYING DIRECTORS

Should members of nonprofit healthcare organizations' boards be paid director's fees? This issue generates considerable debate, and there is likely no one-size-fits-all answer.

Several authors have reviewed the pros and cons of compensating directors, including Alexander (1990), Pointer and Ewell (1994), Johnson and Johnson (1994), Bowen (1994), Hadelman and Orlikoff (1999), and Hupfield (2000). Few studies or surveys have been completed lately to assess how many healthcare organizations pay their directors, and little has been written about the results for those organizations that do. The few available studies (Clark Consulting 2003; Hoffman et al. 1989; Wyatt Company 1986) indicate somewhere between 12 and 25 percent of the hospitals and systems in the United States compensate their directors. The NACD (2010b) survey of nonprofit corporations showed that almost 24 percent pay directors. The American Hospital Association does not track which of their member hospitals pay directors.

Some observers believe that healthcare boards that compensate their directors pay a retainer as well as remuneration for each meeting attended. Although few members may need the money, just knowing they are being compensated seems to raise their level of conscientiousness, particularly about attendance and meeting preparation. Other means of compensating directors include deferred compensation, healthcare benefits, or life insurance. Officers and chairs of committees are sometimes paid an additional amount. Some hospitals or health systems may consider board compensation as much of an investment in their future success as the compensation packages paid to the executive management team.

Some anecdotal evidence indicates that healthcare organizations compensating their boards have had a good experience recruiting new board members, have high attendance at board meetings, and have an easier time conducting self-assessment surveys.

It is strongly recommended boards should at least consider paying director's fees. Generally, however, board members themselves will not bring up the subject, so it should be raised by the chair or the CEO. The range of compensation for hospitals and health systems varies, with a little higher pay for a health system board than the board of a hospital. A range of $6,000 to $15,000 (retainer and per meeting fee) appears to be the most common amount. The revised IRS Form 990 may provide more than anecdotal information in this area.

To expedite such a discussion, Exhibit 2.1 includes the most common pros and cons about the issue.

## STRUCTURE OF THE ANNUAL RETREAT

Whoever coined the saying "It wasn't raining when Noah built the ark" may well have been advising someone to schedule a board retreat before a crisis occurs. If the hospital board chair or CEO waits until a crisis occurs, it will probably be too late to accomplish much in that high-stress environment. All boards should already be in the habit of having an annual retreat; if not, this deficit should be remedied as soon as possible. Planning the annual board retreat is usually the responsibility of the governance committee; the goal should be to get the board members out of their home base to a place where they can comfortably discuss the key issues not normally covered during a regular board meeting.

A board retreat can provide an opportunity for planning; a chance to refocus on fundamentals; a vehicle for team building and strengthening trust and relationships among board members; and a venue to conduct the self-assessment of the board. It

**Exhibit 2.1: The Pros and Cons of Paying Board Directors**

**Why Directors Should Be Paid**
- Compensating board members, regardless of the amount, increases attendance and participation at meetings. Board members also appear to prepare better for meetings. Whatever their motivation, board members do not want to give the appearance of being paid for work they do not do. Members who do not want to be compensated may donate the money back to the organization and receive a tax deduction.
- Most chairs of compensated boards view compensation as a way to recognize board members' efforts, rather than as an incentive for better performance. Compensating a director sends a clear message her work is important to a board whose work is important. It is a tangible recognition of the value of the board member's time in preparing for and attending meetings. The message also tells board members the organization wants their full attention and is willing to compensate them to achieve that.
- Paying board members does not necessarily diminish the community-oriented and charitable mission of the hospital. Compensation may allow participation by community representatives who might not otherwise be able to afford to serve, thus broadening representation and diversity on the board.
- A growing number of CEOs report having trouble, especially in the past five years, recruiting qualified board members. Competition for good board members has increased in many communities, and the hospital may well be in a contest with organizations that pay their board members. Some CEOs contend compensation helps tip the balance for some board candidates. Candidates rarely ask if compensation is part of board service and usually are surprised—and delighted—to know it is. It may also help some board candidates know they will receive at least a token amount for the time or money they might otherwise lose while serving on the board.
- Compensating board members allows more flexibility in recruitment. A hospital may need to move outside its immediate community to find desired expertise. It can be difficult to recruit those individuals if they are expected to pay their own expenses to participate in board activities.
- Compensating directors of nonprofit healthcare organizations can help discourage the feeling that whatever they do or don't do is fine, because after all, they are "only" volunteers.
- Some CEOs believe board compensation makes management feel more comfortable calling on the board to ask for help between meetings.
- Paying directors of publicly traded companies is well established. Compensating a corporate director sends a clear message the board's work is important and the individual's time is valuable. If this is true for these corporations, then why would it not be true for hospitals or health systems, which may be the largest employer in a community or may be a billion-dollar business more complex than many publicly traded companies?

## Why Directors Should Not Be Paid

- One school of thought indicates the essence of voluntary trusteeship precludes compensation—that is, volunteers get far greater satisfaction from their accomplishments, and they will make a greater contribution, because they function for purely altruistic reasons rather than monetary ones.
- Board members may worry about the appearance of a conflict of interest if they receive payment for their services.
- Compensating board members introduces an economic variable that may interfere with the board's ability to objectively conduct an honest and complete self-assessment program.
- Some boards fear they could lose their indemnification privileges as volunteer directors if they are paid. Most state laws make it clear directors are expected to act in good faith within the scope of their official action and duties, but because the laws are so vague otherwise, any challenges will likely be decided by the courts.
- There appears to be no scientifically based evidence compensation improves recruitment or performance of trustees of nonprofit boards. As noted earlier, anecdotal evidence suggests compensating directors improves attendance, but it has not been scientifically proven.
- The relatively small amount many hospitals or health systems could or would pay may not make much difference in attracting and retaining the most qualified individuals.
- Although the compensation might be small, many directors feel the appearance of directors paying themselves sends the wrong message to the community about the board's concern for healthcare costs.

can also provide time to focus on potential problems before they erupt or to seize an opportunity before it is lost.

A board retreat is no longer considered a luxury; it has become an essential activity the board must engage in. The hospital or health system's budget should include a line item for board education activities, including the retreat, sending the message that board development is a priority.

## Making a Board Retreat Successful

- **Obtain obvious leadership support.** A board retreat will not be successful unless it is obvious the retreat is considered to be very important to the chair, the CEO, and other officers of the board. The chair must make it clear the retreat is a priority, and 100 percent attendance is expected.

- **Obtain board input in the planning process.** Board members are more likely to support the need for a retreat and participate actively if they are involved in the planning. Many governance committees find it helpful to send a brief questionnaire to the full board, asking about subjects to cover. The committee should accommodate all responses if possible, particularly if any patterns emerge.

- **Schedule the event with adequate notice.** If the chair expects to get 100 percent attendance at the retreat, it should be scheduled at least five to six months in advance. The governance committee, in its preplanning questionnaire, should ask the board for input on the best time for the retreat—weekday or weekend—and for information about already scheduled plans that would preclude attendance. Every effort should be made to accommodate these responses and to plan the event around conflicts.

- **Be clear about who should attend.** If the board will be addressing sensitive or confidential matters, participation should be limited to directors. If the purpose of the retreat is to look at future options for the organization and review certain types of data and presentations, the event can be a leadership retreat appropriate for key staff to attend. In general, most board members are reluctant to say what they really think about any controversial issues in front of nonboard members. Just be clear about what is to be accomplished and what issues are to be discussed before deciding if it is a board retreat or a leadership retreat.

- **Select the right location.** The event should be a true retreat. The board needs to get away from the place where normal business is conducted. The location does not have to be a great distance away nor expensive, but board members must be far enough from home that they will not check in regularly with their staffs or leave early to return to their offices. They need to be where they can comfortably get to know each other better and focus on the issues in detail without distractions. One of the duties of the committee planning the retreat is to explore different locations, such as country inns and resorts, campgrounds or lodges at state or national parks, spiritual retreat centers, university conference centers, or corporate retreat centers.

- **Design the agenda carefully.** The best retreats tend to be built around a single, clearly defined theme. These retreats focus on one or two issues of importance to the board, and everyone understands the objectives. The agenda should not be too ambitious; better to have ample time to do good work on one issue than for the group to leave feeling frustrated because they could not deal with overly grand expectations. Make sure the issue or theme is not something that can be handled at a routine board meeting. At least half of the time should be allocated for the board members to fully discuss the issues.

This discussion will let the board members get to know and understand each other. Most board members will not speak up if they feel there is no time for their comments. Excellent outside speakers will not make up for the opportunity for board members to discuss an issue among themselves.

- **Select the facilitator carefully.** Having the CEO or board chair facilitate will ensure a disastrous retreat. The CEO and the chair cannot participate fully in addition to running the meeting, and it is unfair to ask them to try. Having the usual authority figure in charge can also inhibit discussion and allow the retreat to fall into the pattern of a regular board meeting. Retaining the services of an experienced consultant to facilitate will keep the discussion moving forward, ensure everyone takes the opportunity to participate, and allow the CEO and chair to contribute. An objective facilitator can more easily prevent the board from getting off track during discussions of difficult subjects and can make sure conclusions are reached in an appropriate time. The board chair or CEO can lead part of the discussion, depending on the issue, but a facilitator will make the retreat more successful and satisfactory for everyone.

- **Plan adequate social time.** The retreat schedule must allow time for board members to get to know each other socially. They will function better as a board and enjoy working together more if they come together as a team through social interaction. Even within small communities, board members do not necessarily travel in the same circles. Public boards, such as those involved with district or county hospitals, have an even greater need to become acquainted as individuals; these boards are not self-perpetuating and cannot decide who will be appointed by the county commissioners or elected by the public. Allowing adequate social time may very well be the most important part of a board retreat. If board members learn to know, respect, and get along with one other, they just might learn to govern better together.

- **Develop an action plan for handling follow-up.** In general, boards take no votes and make no official decisions at a retreat. The retreat format should be designed to encourage full participation and creative thinking. Although conclusions should be reached so that no discussion is left hanging, formal votes should be left for subsequent business meetings. At the very least, the facilitator should be able to summarize the discussion in such a way that attendees can all agree with the result. That summary should ideally lead to development of an action plan with timetables so that the board agrees on the next steps. The summary and action plan process can help prevent individual board members from feeling like they attended different retreats. The post-retreat interval can be used for staff or committees to tie up loose ends.

# BOARD SELF-ASSESSMENT PROCESS AND SAMPLE ASSESSMENT TOOL

Not too long ago, it was unheard of for boards to even think about the need to do a self-assessment, let alone to do one. However, as with so many other things in healthcare, that is changing, and recent upheavals in the corporate world compel any responsible board to take a closer look at how it functions. Many regulatory or quasi-regulatory bodies in both the nonprofit and for-profit sectors, including The Joint Commission and the New York Stock Exchange, require boards to complete a regular self-assessment process.

Boards that complete a self-assessment program seem to quickly solve many of their problems, even some that have plagued them for years. Self-assessments provide a way for a board to fulfill its commitment to quality, for itself as well as for the hospital or health system as a whole.

Although there are many ways a board can complete the process, having an objective outside consultant coordinate the project avoids any conflict of interest or appearance of conflict of interest, and board members seem to feel freer to share their thoughts. However, it is better for the hospital board to do something—including completing the process internally—than to do nothing at all. Exhibit 2.2 is an example of a self-assessment process used by several hospitals.

## Step One

Before a scheduled retreat where the board is going to do its self-evaluation, send a survey tool to board members for anonymous response. Exhibit 2.2 provides 30 sample questions that have been regularly refined and updated. A board may add specific questions relating to a particular environment or situation or delete questions considered less relevant. Set a deadline to encourage members to respond in a timely manner.

## Step Two

The consultant tabulates the answers and identifies those areas where responses show a significant variance.

Interestingly, most boards appear to be in general agreement on 22 to 25 of the questions—that is, they *strongly agree* or *agree*, and one or two members will be in the *somewhat disagree* column. However, the responses on four to six of the questions will

## BOARD OF DIRECTORS
## SAMPLE SELF-ASSESSMENT

Please check one answer for each question/statement. Results will be tabulated to reflect how board members feel about each question as a group. Responses are anonymous, and no individual response is ever identified. The goal is to determine how the board relates to these items *as a group*. **If you are not sure of an answer, please leave it blank.**

Please return by: _____

Please email, fax, or mail your answers to: _____

1. Each board member knows and is comfortable with the hospital's current mission statement.
   Rating: _____strongly agree _____agree _____somewhat disagree _____disagree

2. Proposals brought before the board are evaluated to ensure they are consistent with the hospital's mission, vision, goals, and objectives.
   Rating: _____strongly agree _____agree _____somewhat disagree _____disagree

3. The board has adopted a strategic plan, which is reviewed regularly.
   Rating: _____strongly agree _____agree _____somewhat disagree _____disagree

4. The board generally understands the concept of "cooptition," whereby physicians cooperate with the hospital at times and compete with the hospital in other situations.
   Rating: _____strongly agree _____agree _____somewhat disagree _____disagree

5. Participation of physicians and/or nurses is sought in the governance process to assist the board in fulfilling its responsibilities regarding the provision of quality patient care.
   Rating: _____strongly agree _____agree _____somewhat disagree _____disagree

6. Membership on the board is open to physicians or other health professionals who function as regular board members and who have been selected by the same criteria as other members of the board.
   Rating: _____strongly agree _____agree _____somewhat disagree _____disagree

7. The board appoints individuals to the medical staff based on clearly established criteria and a medical staff recommendation.
   Rating: _____strongly agree _____agree _____somewhat disagree _____disagree

8. The board reviews comparative statistical data on the quality of the hospital's clinical services and patient care and sets targets to ensure improvement.
   Rating: _____strongly agree _____agree _____somewhat disagree _____disagree

*(continued)*

9. The board reviews and adopts an annual budget, setting revenue and expense targets, and considers regular reports during the year to determine ompliance.
   Rating: _____strongly agree _____agree _____somewhat disagree _____disagree

10. The board approves specific parameters on items such as debt, liquidity, return on investment, and other financial ratios to provide early warning signals of financial problems.
    Rating: _____strongly agree _____agree _____somewhat disagree _____disagree

11. The board adopts a long-term capital expenditure plan that estimates projected sources, costs, and uses of future funding for buildings and equipment.
    Rating: _____strongly agree _____agree _____somewhat disagree _____disagree

12. Board policies and criteria for the selection of new members are clearly defined and followed to ensure continuing leadership and accessibility of needed knowledge and skills.
    Rating: _____strongly agree _____agree _____somewhat disagree _____disagree

13. The board evaluates its performance to determine its effectiveness and to identify needed skills and knowledge for board continuity and growth.
    Rating: _____strongly agree _____agree _____somewhat disagree _____disagree

14. The board periodically reviews its size, structure, committees, materials it receives for meetings, tenure of members, officers, and committee chairpersons.
    Rating: _____strongly agree _____agree _____somewhat disagree _____disagree

15. The board or its executive committee conducts an evaluation of the CEO each year using specific criteria agreed upon in advance with the CEO.
    Rating: _____strongly agree _____agree _____somewhat disagree _____disagree

16. The board understands and values the difference between the board's policymaking role and the CEO's management role.
    Rating: _____strongly agree _____agree _____somewhat disagree _____disagree

17. The board communicates effectively with the CEO regarding goals and expectations.
    Rating: _____strongly agree _____agree _____somewhat disagree _____disagree

18. The board supports the CEO in his/her relationships with the medical staff.
    Rating: _____strongly agree _____agree _____somewhat disagree _____disagree

19. The board has a policy regarding identification and resolution of real or perceived conflicts of interest by its members and/or the administrative staff.
    Rating: _____strongly agree _____agree _____somewhat disagree _____disagree

20. All members of the board have job descriptions and understand their responsibilities, roles, and duties.
    Rating: _____strongly agree _____agree _____somewhat disagree _____disagree

21. All members of the board participate in an orientation program and continuing education.
Rating: _____strongly agree _____agree _____somewhat disagree _____disagree

22. The board regularly reviews data about the medical staff to ensure future staffing will be adequate regarding numbers and needed specialties.
Rating: _____strongly agree _____agree _____somewhat disagree _____disagree

23. The chairperson ensures all board members have equal opportunity to participate, time is not monopolized by a few, and agenda items are appropriately handled following adequate discussion.
Rating: _____strongly agree _____agree _____somewhat disagree _____disagree

24. The board has a written job description for the position of board chair.
Rating: _____strongly agree _____agree _____somewhat disagree _____disagree

25. The board has a clear chair selection and succession process, which is used.
Rating: _____strongly agree _____agree _____somewhat disagree _____disagree

26. The board has a position of chair-elect, or its equivalent, which is filled one year before the individual assumes the office of chair.
Rating: _____strongly agree _____agree _____somewhat disagree _____disagree

27. The chair's performance is evaluated by the board.
Rating: _____strongly agree _____agree _____somewhat disagree _____disagree

28. The board reviews and discusses emerging healthcare innovations and changes in healthcare technology as part of the continuing education programs that occur at board meetings or during board retreats.
Rating: _____strongly agree _____agree _____somewhat disagree _____disagree

29. The board represents the hospital to the total community and does not advocate for any particular constituency or geographical area.
Rating: _____strongly agree _____agree _____somewhat disagree _____disagree

30. Despite individual disagreements and compromises, the board consistently reaches decisions that allow it to move forward in a unified fashion.
Rating: _____strongly agree _____agree _____somewhat disagree _____disagree

Comments: _____

_____

_____

_____

_____

usually be all over the place, and on rare occasions, the entire board will respond with *disagree* or *strongly disagree* on one of them. These are the questions the board needs to spend time addressing, and the consultant can expedite that process.

In one example, board members' responses to four questions had quite different answers. Using a "shorthand version" of the questions as given in Exhibit 2.2, the differing responses to questions 2, 13, 25, and 28 are shown in Exhibit 2.3. There were 15 board members and 15 responses.

## Step Three

Following tabulation, the consultant needs to help the board address the results. How can the board most effectively discuss these four questions to more closely agree on them?

One technique is to divide the board into groups of three to five members. The four challenged statements from the survey are rephrased into questions for each group to analyze.

For example, item 2 on the survey, "Proposals brought before the board are evaluated to ensure they are consistent with the hospital's mission, vision, goals and objectives," becomes, "What can we as board do to ensure our decisions are consistent with our mission, vision, goals, and objectives?"

Item 13 on the survey, "The board evaluates its performance to determine its effectiveness and to identify needed skills and knowledge for board continuity and growth," becomes, "What can we as a board do to more effectively evaluate our own performance and the performance of each board member?"

**Exhibit 2.3: Summary of Responses (Board of Directors Self-Assessment)**

| Question | Strongly Agree | Agree | Somewhat Disagree | Disagree |
|---|---|---|---|---|
| 2. Consistent with mission | 3/15 (20%) | 2/15 (13%) | 6/15 (40%) | 4/15 (27%) |
| 13. Board performance | 2/15 (13%) | 6/15 (40%) | 3/15 (20%) | 4/15 (27%) |
| 25. Chair selection process | 4/15 (27%) | 2/15 (13%) | 5/15 (33%) | 4/15 (27%) |
| 28. Board reviews technology | 4/15 (27%) | 6/15 (40%) | 2/15 (13%) | 3/15 (20%) |

Item 25 on the survey, "The board has and uses a clear chair selection and succession process," becomes, "What do we need to do to improve our chair selection and succession process?"

Item 28, "The board reviews and discusses emerging health care innovations and changes in healthcare technology as part of the continuing education programs that occur at board meetings or during board retreats," becomes, "How can we as a board improve our knowledge of new healthcare technology and other healthcare innovations?"

Each group is then given a question to review, discuss, and make suggestions for solutions. The suggested solutions are then put in an envelope and passed to the next group, which will repeat the process without looking at the prior group's suggestions. The questions continue around the groups in this fashion until they reach the last group. This final group will review what the prior groups have suggested, add its own thoughts if they have not already been covered, and then craft a final recommendation for presentation to the entire board.

Using this technique, each board member has the opportunity to help identify problem areas and contribute to solutions; all board members become involved in creating viable solutions; and before the retreat is over, the board has worked as a team to move forward. Work done using this technique provides a sense of accomplishment, with no board member feeling left out or personally challenged, and it sets a great precedent for handling future challenges.


## DEALING WITH A DISRUPTIVE OR INATTENTIVE BOARD MEMBER

Not much has been written about how a board should deal with a disruptive or inattentive board member, mainly because it is a sensitive issue. There is a difference between disruptive and inattentive. Inattentive board members miss board meetings, board retreats, or specially held meetings (or show up late and leave early); do not read materials before meetings; or do not contribute to discussions. Disruptive board members dominate board discussions, ignore the agenda, force discussion on extraneous issues, are offensive in board discussions, and in general are difficult and inconsiderate people.

Disruptive board members can and often do have a negative impact on the board's overall effectiveness and efficiency. Any behavior that interferes significantly with the process of governance should be considered disruptive and requires attention.

If the board uses annual performance appraisals (see Appendixes 3 and 4), the disruptive behavior should be well documented and can be used as a basis for a discussion with the offending board member. The board chair and CEO (or the chair of the governance committee) must meet with this board member to clearly but firmly explain that his behavior will no longer be tolerated, and if it continues, they expect his resignation.

Who should be involved in a meeting with the disruptive board member? There should be two people meeting with the board member; one should always be the board chair. The other person should be the CEO or the chair of the governance committee, depending on the individual hospital board structure and culture. There will be more impact on the board member when two people meet with her than one. The overall effectiveness and efficiency of the board comes first and if that requires demanding a resignation, so be it.

With the inattentive board member who does not seem fully engaged in the business of the board, problems such as attendance and other disengaged behaviors can be addressed by the board chair or the governance committee during the annual performance appraisal.

Both the disruptive member and the inattentive member need to clearly understand they must change the offending behaviors or resign. Exhibit 2.4 is a sample letter a board chair might write to a board member who needs to resign because of attendance problems.

---

**Exhibit 2.4: Sample Board Member Removal Letter**

*Dear Errol:*

*This letter is not easy to write. You have been an important player on our hospital board, and we are grateful for your energy and vision.*

*As we discussed during our meeting last week, the past year has been difficult for you since you began a new job that takes you out of town a lot. It has become increasingly apparent other responsibilities make it difficult for you to be present for our board meetings or to take an active role on committee assignments.*

*You know how necessary it is for this hospital to have the active interest and participation of each member. Therefore, I hope you will understand my request that you resign before the end of your term to make room for someone who has more time.*

*We all hope the day will come when your other activities will allow you to join the board again. We will miss you.*

*Sincerely,*

*Alison Knight*
*Board Chair*

---

Again, the board chair and chair of the governance committee need to remember the overall effectiveness and efficiency of the board come first, and that may mean requesting some resignations from the board.

## References

Alexander, J. 1990. *The Changing Character of Hospital Governance*. Chicago: American Hospital Association.

Biggs, E. 2001. "Terminating Board Term Limits." *Trustee* 54 (2): 21–23.

———. 2000. "Selecting the Right Physician for Your Board." *Trustee* 53 (9): 22–23.

Bowen, W. G. 1994. *Inside the Boardroom*. New York: Wiley.

Clark Consulting (now Integrated Healthcare Strategies). 2003. "Healthcare Board of Directors Compensation Survey." Minneapolis, MN: Clark Consulting.

Hadelman, J., and J. Orlikoff. 1999. "Get Real. Professional Governing Boards Must Happen if Hospitals and Systems Are to Survive." *Modern Healthcare* 29 (41): 32.

Health Care Advisory Board. 1996. "The Rising Tide." Washington, DC: Health Care Advisory Board.

Hoffman, J. R., T. C. Hermann, D. R. Rich, R. L. Johnson, and S. L. Gill. 1989. "Compensation of Hospital Governing Boards: A National Survey." *Healthcare Executive* 4 (3): 34–35.

Hupfield, S. F. 2000. "Board Compensation: The Time Is Now." *Trustee* 53 (1): 28–30.

Integrated Healthcare Strategies. 2009. "2009 Compensation Survey." Minneapolis, MN: Integrated Health Strategies.

Johnson, E. A., and R. L. Johnson. 1994. *New Dynamics for Hospital Boards*. Chicago: Health Administration Press.

McEvoy, G., and W. Cascio. 1989. "Cumulative Evidence of the Relationship Between Employee Age and Job Performance." *Journal of Applied Psychology* 75 (1): 11–17.

National Association of Corporate Directors (NACD). 2010a. "2009 Public Company Governance Survey." Washington, DC: National Association of Corporate Directors.

———. 2010b. "2009 NACD Nonprofit Governance Survey." Washington, DC: National Association of Corporate Directors.

Orlikoff, J. E., and M. Totten. 2008. "The New Board Chair." *Healthcare Executive* January/February 23: 56–58.

Pointer, D. D., and C. M. Ewell. 1994. *Really Governing: How Health Systems and Hospital Boards Can Make More of a Difference.* Albany, NY: Delmar.

Prybil, L. 2008. "Governance in Nonprofit Community Health Systems," 11. Chicago: The Center for Healthcare Governance.

Rhodes, S. 1983. "Age-Related Differences in Work Attitudes and Behavior: A Review and Conceptual Analysis." *Psychological Bulletin* 93 (2): 328–67.

Schaie, K. W. 1996. "Intellectual Development in Adulthood." In *Handbook of the Psychology of Aging,* edited by J. E. Birren and K. W. Schaie, 4th edition. San Diego: Academic Press.

Wyatt Company. 1986. "Practices of Boards of Directors/Trustees in the Health Care Industry." Fort Lee, NJ: Executive Compensation Services.

# CHAPTER THREE

# How to Build Your Board

## SELECTING NEW MEMBERS

If new board members are identified and selected carefully, the subsequent work of the board should flow smoothly and creatively for the benefit of the hospital or health system. If members are selected with little thought or research, the board

- misses the opportunity to fill a talent void,
- runs the risk of adding a difficult personality to the mix, and
- may bring on someone who is not actually interested in the organization at all.

The governance committee should use specific criteria for those it recommends for board membership.

It can be difficult for a hospital to compete and thrive in today's environment with the wrong people on the board. Some of Jim Collins's research in his book *Good to Great* (2001) relates directly to how important it is for boards of directors to select the right people. In his research, Collins found the great companies

> ...[f]irst get the right people on the bus, the wrong people off the bus, and the right people in the right seats—and then they figure out where to drive it. The old adage that people are your most important asset turns out to be wrong; people are not your most important asset. The right people are.

Collins also found people in the great companies clearly loved what they did, largely because they loved with whom they did it.

These same concepts work for hospital and health system boards as well. Each board is likely to have some of its own specific criteria. However, the following general criteria are provided for overall consideration; they can offer the governance committee a process for making recommendations.

## RECRUITING FOR DIVERSITY

While people often consider diversity of race, gender, or ethnic background, for hospital and health system boards, diversity goes beyond those categories. The skill sets, interests, and backgrounds of potential new members should be different from those of current board members but still aligned with the strategic direction of the hospital.

### Experience

Board experience of some type is important. The local chamber of commerce can be a useful resource for those who are or have been on the boards of organizations in the area. The healthcare learning curve can be quite steep, so it is best to identify potential board members who already have a reasonable idea about functioning in a board role—they won't have to learn two new roles simultaneously.

### Achievement

Prospective board members should be individuals who have accomplished something. It could be in building a business, serving on the board of an organization that provides a needed service to the community, doing something that resulted in personal recognition, being an outstanding teacher in the local high school or college, or accomplishing anything that denotes personal achievement.

## Occupation and Skill

Boards go through stages where their attention needs to be focused on a specific portion of the hospital's goals and objectives or strategic plan. Accordingly, different skill sets can be needed at different times. The board, or governance committee, should periodically determine what experience and skills would be useful and whether there are holes in the board's knowledge base.

Examples might include someone with in-depth financial skills, or a quality care guru, or perhaps an individual who had worked with a construction or remodeling project might fill a niche. At times, the board may need to look outside the community for the missing expertise, and it is becoming more common for boards to do so. The key is to find individuals who bring something of benefit to the hospital or health system.

## Ability to Be a Team Player

Being on a board is a team sport. People who do not play well with others are usually not good board members. For example, sometimes entrepreneurs have difficulties with teamwork because they are used to acting alone and not delegating. Some surgeons find being a team player difficult because of their training to make quick decisions, see instant results, and be the "captain of the ship."

In a similar fashion, followers or "yes men" may not make the best board members. These individuals frequently offer very little during a discussion, tend not to speak until everyone else has contributed, and then ride in on the coattails of whomever they perceive is leading the group at the time. They bring nothing to the table, and the team derives no benefit from their presence.

## Affluence

Affluence can be a controversial criterion, but one that should not be discounted. Many affluent people have been successful in business and know what it takes to get results. They often have a social conscience, plus the time to spend on a board. Affluent people can frequently resist pressures from medical staffs, employee groups, community groups, or special-interest stakeholder groups. This ability is particularly important in a smaller community where so many people know one other. Wealth alone should not disqualify anyone from board consideration.

## Interest in and Commitment to the Organization

Board members must share an interest in and commitment to the hospital's mission, vision, goals, and objectives, and the governance committee should actively screen board prospects by these measures. Directors of children's hospitals throughout the United States almost always seem to have had a child treated at the hospital or a close relationship with someone who had a child in the hospital. These individuals clearly understand the hospital's mission, believe in it, and are committed to it. Usually, if a children's hospital is having financial difficulties, the mission of caring for sick children comes first, and how it is to be funded comes second. Between effective fundraising, adherence to the mission, and strategic affiliations, children's hospitals can survive and sometimes flourish. This is not to say boards should lead an organization to a financial calamity. Rather, individuals on the board must know and support the hospital's mission to advance the organization in a fiscally sound manner.

## Personal Qualities

Look for personal qualities that will make the individual a good board member. Does she have high integrity? Does he show compassion? Is she a good listener? Are high morals apparent? Is he intelligent? Will she make decisions based on facts and not emotion? These qualities will be important if the hospital faces difficult times or hard decisions and the board must speak with one voice.

## Objectivity

Members serve on the board to function as a team for the benefit of the organization, its stakeholders, and the community it serves, not to advocate for social causes or represent a particular constituency such as a group of employees, special interest groups, or geographic areas. The board needs good, objective members; whether they happen to be minorities, nurses, physicians, bankers, or trapeze artists should be of little consequence.

The only individual on the board or attending board meetings who represents a constituency by virtue of her office is the president of the medical staff. This individual speaks for the medical staff, and everyone else at the table knows and expects it. They would, in fact, be surprised if she did otherwise. However, the governance committee should strive to determine if objectivity could be a problem with any potential candidate.

## Receptivity to Training and Evaluation

Boards should seek out members who are receptive to training and self-evaluation. The director who arrives on the board knowing everything frequently stalls the board's progress. The healthcare industry is complex; just because someone knows a particular industry does not mean that knowledge carries over to healthcare. Specific knowledge sets pertain to reimbursement, medical staff relationships, licensure of personnel, and quality measurements. Board members must continually educate themselves about such issues and the changes that affect the hospital.

Board members must also be receptive to opportunities to do not only a regular board self-assessment but to look objectively at what contributions they are making to the hospital as individuals.

## Willingness to Devote Time

The world's greatest board members are useless if they do not have the time to read their materials and attend meetings. The hospital or healthcare system is, in many instances, the largest corporation in a community, having the most employees and the largest revenue base and thus requiring the most talented board members available. But those members must have the time to contribute. A board cannot afford to have letterhead or ornamental directors.

## SELECTING THE RIGHT PHYSICIANS FOR THE BOARD

(Adapted from *Trustee*, Vol. 53, No. 9, by permission, October 2000. Copyright 2000, by Health Forum, Inc.)

Hospital boards should consider having two or three physicians as board members. Physicians can enhance the board's ability to make good decisions for the benefit of the community and the quality of care available to patients.

The placement of the right physicians on a hospital board of directors could very well be one of the most relevant sections of this book; increased attention to conflict-of-interest issues should require governance committees to look carefully at how physicians are appointed to the board.* The new Form 990 hospitals must file with the IRS has changed significantly regarding who is considered an "independent" board member, and it requires a majority of the directors to be independent. The basic rule: As long as the physician is not being compensated in any amount by the hospital as an employee, or more than $10,000 as an independent contractor, or there is no reportable direct or indirect business transaction between the physician and the hospital, then the physician board member can be counted as independent on the Form 990.

## Mandated Representational Board Seats for Medical Staff

Boards should consider eliminating the automatic voting board seat for the elected chief or president of the medical staff. As Karma Bass (2008) points out, this practice puts the physician in an untenable position if disputes arise between medical staff physicians and the hospital. This seems to be happening more today than at any time in the past. The automatic board seat can hinder both effective governance and effective hospital–physician relations.

Because the president of the medical staff is elected by the medical staff, she represents the interests of the medical staff constituency. However, all board members are required to make decisions in the best interests of the hospital, even if the decision disadvantages a particular group or constituency. This legal mandate, under the fiduciary duty of loyalty, places the medical staff representative/board member in the impossible situation of having a legal master—the board—and an implied master—the medical staff.

The old model of automatic medical staff involvement in governance obviously will not work anymore. The board should determine if it needs participation from one or two other objective members who happen to be physicians. The best solution for the hospital board may be to give the medical staff president a nonvoting seat at the table and find another physician to serve on the board through the usual board nomination and recruitment process. Unfortunately, whether an individual physician is the right one for the board at any given time may not be known until he is already on the board. However, if a good selection process is in place, and the governance committee follows the process it has developed, the uncertainty is more likely to be avoided.

How should these other potential physician board members be selected for consideration?

## Deciding Which Types of Physicians Are Not Eligible

Concern about conflicts of interest appears on most hospital boards' lists of issues. It also is high on the lists of the IRS, the media, regulators, and legislators, to name a few interested parties. Boards that participate in self-assessment programs are particularly interested in this topic; therefore, boards that are selecting physician members should pay particular attention.

Although exceptions sometimes exist, the board governance committee should eliminate all hospital-based physicians from consideration. This generally includes pathologists, radiologists, anesthesiologists, hospitalists, intensivists, medical directors, emergency department physicians, or any physician who is on the hospital's payroll or who has a contract with the hospital. Why?

As an example, it is difficult for the hospital CEO to recommend a particular piece of expensive equipment not be purchased for radiology when the radiologist is a member of the board, or worse yet, is the chair or an officer of the board. Likewise, when an anesthesiologist comes to the CEO and wants his group to have an "exclusive contract" with the hospital but does not want the group to be prevented from providing anesthesia services to a competing surgery center, that poses problems for the hospital if the anesthesiologist is on the board. Further, when physicians who are on the hospital's payroll are also on the board, it is virtually impossible for the CEO to negotiate salary or salary increases, either for the physician board member (who is her boss) or for herself. These obvious conflicts of interest can be avoided if such physicians are not seated on the board in the first place.

Any one of the physicians mentioned here may also be put in a difficult position if other members of that physician's group put pressure on him to push their agenda items or proposals.

In a small, four-hospital system, the governance committee was about to recommend to the board that they make a pathologist the new chair of the system board. The pathologist had been on the board, was a nice person, had helped merge the first two hospitals in the system, had been a good board member, and was respected by everyone. At the board meeting, a director who happened to be the CEO of a local company and who happened to play golf with the pathologist asked if he was the only one who saw a huge conflict-of-interest problem. The pathologist's group held an exclusive contract with the hospital system to provide all the pathology services to the system. The board member asked if the IRS, attorney general, or donors might think it was strange for this individual to be the board chair. The board decided to hold off on the nomination and asked the governance committee to draw up guidelines regarding physician board service and board chair selection. After studying the matter thoroughly and objectively, the governance committee recommended that any physicians who had a contract with the system would not be eligible for board membership.

More and more physicians are in groups being acquired by hospitals or healthcare systems, or are going into specialties such as hospitalists, which make them ineligible for board membership. At a hospital board retreat, a board member mentioned that any physician who had a contract with the hospital was not eligible to be on the board. The hospital CEO noted 50 percent of the physicians on the medical staff had some sort of contract with the hospital. The solution was easy: The board does not consider that 50 percent, but does consider the other 50 percent if it wants physicians from the community on the board.

## Deciding Which Types of Physicians Are Eligible

The board's governance committee should determine which types of physicians are least likely to have potential conflicts of interests. These categories would include those not employed by the hospital, such as primary care physicians (e.g., family practitioners, internists, obstetricians, pediatricians). Other candidates could include cardiologists, oncologists, infectious disease specialists, pulmonologists, general surgeons, orthopedic surgeons, and urologists. Many CEOs prefer to have primary care physicians on the board because they are less dependent on the hospital for their livelihoods, and they may support decisions that are medically necessary instead of just financially feasible.

The governance committee should remember: Do not ask the medical staff for recommendations! The medical staff will be represented at board meetings by their president, who is the main spokesperson for that group of stakeholders. The board does not need two or three more physicians also representing the medical staff.

## Selecting the Physician Candidate

The board, through its governance committee, should have a methodical process of identifying specific physician candidates for the board using similar criteria for selecting physician board members as it uses for other members.

### Experience
Physicians who have had no other board experience should not be selected. The hospital is too important to the community to provide a learning ground for novices. The resumes of all members of the medical staff should be on file at the hospital and should be current, as all members of the medical staff have to be reappointed regularly. Resumes of physicians who would not have a conflict of interest should be reviewed to ascertain if the physicians are on or have recently served on any other boards, such as corporations, professional associations, churches, Boy Scouts, or other community-based groups.

Physicians who have served on other boards should understand the requirements of a board member, particularly the importance of fiduciary responsibilities and the duties of care, loyalty, and obedience.

## Achievement

The resumes should also provide information about achievements of eligible physicians. Have they been elected to any offices by the local, state, or national medical society or by other groups on whose boards they have served? Have they received awards from those groups or from their peers? Have they achieved something or been recognized for an activity outside of medicine? On what kinds of hospital committees have they served? Do they bring other knowledge or experiences to the board?

## Management Skills

To maintain their present income levels in today's unsettled environment, physicians need creativity, financial knowledge, and management skills. Many physicians today are getting MBAs or attending short-term management courses sponsored by professional associations or universities. Has the physician done anything to improve her management skills? What kind of continuing education programs has she attended in the past five years? Is the physician the managing partner of her group practice? These skills can be put to good use for the benefit of the hospital.

## Ability to Be a Team Player

Serving effectively on a board is not an individual sport. The board's governance committee should look for indications the physician is or can be a team player. Some clinical specialties tend to stress teamwork more than others, but most physicians are not trained to be team players. The hierarchical nature of the clinical training model does not prepare physicians to share decision-making authority with nonphysicians, and sometimes not even with other physicians. They are taught to look at a problem, review all the options, make a decision, and see if it was good or bad based on outcomes. All of this happens quickly. CEOs and boards may not know for several years if their decision was good or bad. A physician who cannot adapt to this environment may become frustrated and lose his usefulness to the board.

## Personal Qualities

Some personal qualities the governance committee should consider include intelligence, compassion, listening skills, and willingness to compromise. The physician must have high moral and ethical standards, and integrity is an absolute must.

## Objectivity

Board members must come to meetings with open minds and without personal agendas, willing to put the welfare of the hospital first in all deliberations. Look for physician candidates who will be objective. No board member should represent a specific constituency. (The president of the medical staff is the only exception.) However, professionals such as physicians tend to identify with peers and similarly trained individuals rather than with an organization. Physicians who go through the hospital board selection process should be sensitive to the need to be objective. The use of job descriptions for all board members helps maintain their objectivity.

## Receptivity to Training and Education

Although physicians are receptive to medical continuing education and training, make sure the physician candidate will be receptive to board education programs. The physician's rugged individualist mentality can make it challenging for physician board members to continue learning about governance.

## Special Considerations

Boards of smaller hospitals in rural communities sometimes have difficulty finding physician board members because of the small number of physicians on the medical staff or in the community. If the hospital has six physicians on the medical staff who live in the community and they belong to two different practice groups, it can be politically tough to select one of them to be a board member (in addition to the president of the medical staff). Selecting a physician from the same group as the medical staff president could leave the board open to charges of favoritism, while selecting a physician from the competing group might result in a lack of cooperation on certain issues. Such boards may wish to consider inviting a physician from another noncompeting community to sit on the board or looking for a retired physician.

It may be difficult for some hospitals to have physicians as board members. In district hospitals, for example, board members are elected by the community, so the only way to get good physician members on those boards is to convince the right physicians to run for election. Busy physicians may not be willing to do so. Pitting public opinion against the hospital's needs may present challenges that do not appeal to the average physician.

County hospitals have similar difficulties. Usually, the county commissioners appoint the hospital's board of directors, sometimes along political lines. Historically, physicians have not been the most visible people in political circles, so they tend not to be appointed to these positions.

A county or district board that desires physician input may have to mount its own political campaign to either convince qualified physicians to run for elected office or to convince the county commissioners to appoint physicians with the needed expertise.

## CONSIDERING INDIVIDUALS FROM OUTSIDE THE COMMUNITY

More healthcare boards than ever before are looking outside their communities for members (Greene 2010). When a board determines the specific skills or experiences it needs are not available in the community, it makes more sense to broaden the search area than to leave those needs unfilled. Someone from outside the hospital community can often constructively identify and challenge old board and management assumptions much more easily than someone closer to the situation. In general, outside directors fall into the following categories:

1. **Individuals with unique skills.** These individuals may have expertise in risk management, quality and safety, markets or regions new to the organization, special financial skills, or strategic planning. An outside perspective can also push local board members to think in a different way and prioritize differently, such as raising the importance of quality programs and measures to the same level as financial reports. In addition, outside reviewers such as financial ratings agencies look at the quality of an organization's board and management when issuing bonds. Having a few board members with special expertise and geographic reach can strengthen a rating agency's confidence in the organization.

   A good example of using outside board members is Virginia Mason Medical Center in Seattle (Greene 2010). Julie Morath, who is chief quality officer at Vanderbilt University Medical Center in Nashville, is a member of the board of Virginia Mason and travels to Seattle several times a year for board meetings. James Orlikoff, a Chicago-based governance consultant, is also a member of the board and travels to Seattle for meetings. Morath and Orlikoff were asked to serve on this board because they possess particular skill sets that the board had identified as desirable.

   Presbyterian Healthcare Services in Albuquerque has been recruiting directors from outside New Mexico for about ten years and makes a point of having at least one outside director on each of its key boards and committees (Greene 2010). For example, the board sought out a compliance director from another healthcare system to serve on its compliance committee.

2. **Physicians.** A board may feel it needs physician input beyond that provided by the president of the medical staff, but it may not be comfortable adding another physician from the medical staff. If there are only six physicians in town, with three belonging to one group and three to another group, the board may feel more comfortable recruiting a physician from outside the community. Or a community may have only four physicians, all practicing in one group. If that group decides to move procedures out of the hospital, considerable tension will ensue. One solution to these problems is to recruit a physician from a nearby area. The board should make sure the individual is not in competition with physicians on the medical staff or affiliated with a hospital in competition with the board's hospital.

   Some healthcare systems also recruit physicians who have regional or national recognition in areas such as quality assurance. This could be a solution for small communities that lack the expertise locally.

   It is not just smaller hospitals that add physicians from outside the medical staff to the board; Exempla Health, a three-hospital system in Denver, added Dr. William Jessee to the board, and he eventually became chair. Dr. Jessee heads a national association and has extensive experience working with clinical outcome measures—an asset to the board without the pitfalls of possible conflict of interest or competition.

3. **Hospital CEOs.** Some boards have found it helpful to recruit a CEO (or a retired CEO) from a different state or a noncompeting hospital. These individuals can bring knowledge and objectivity to the board and can help the board understand many of the problems facing the average CEO. The outside CEO can also help the board put its own situation in perspective by sharing how similar problems are handled in another location. Most boards and CEOs who have taken this approach seem very satisfied with it and supportive of the idea. Dan Wilford was the CEO of Memorial Hermann Healthcare System in Houston, Texas, when he served on the board of Mobile Infirmary Medical Center in Mobile, Alabama. After retiring from Memorial Hermann, Wilford began serving on the board of St. Joseph's Healthcare System in Orange, California. His experience with organizational structure has proved valuable to many boards.

   The concept of an outside director is limited to for-profit and nonprofit, 501(c)(3) hospitals. Public and district hospitals whose directors are elected cannot take advantage of this option. However, in county hospitals, where the county commissioners appoint the board, it is possible in some areas to appoint an outside director to the board.

Adding board members from outside the community is not a groundswell movement, but a sampling of organizations where the idea has been implemented includes

- Oakwood Healthcare System, Dearborn, Michigan
- Allina Health System, Minneapolis, Minnesota
- Clarian Health Partners, Indianapolis, Indiana
- Exempla Health, Denver, Colorado
- Intermountain Health Care, Salt Lake City, Utah
- Virginia Mason Medical Center, Seattle, Washington
- Presbyterian Healthcare Services, Albuquerque, New Mexico
- St. Joseph's Healthcare System, Orange, California

## EFFECTIVE ORIENTATION FOR NEW BOARD MEMBERS

Each hospital or health system is a unique entity, with its own structure and manner of functioning. Even the most experienced and knowledgeable new board member cannot be expected to arrive knowing those specific components. A well-planned orientation program will help new board members learn their way around, understand their roles, and meet both their own and the board's expectations.

When designing a meaningful orientation program, it is important to ask continuing board members what they know now that they wish they had known when they first joined the board. This information can then be included in the program's design as appropriate. Some continuing members may find such a program to be a welcome refresher course for them as well; therefore, they should not be discouraged from attending, but they should not be allowed to dominate the sessions.

It can be difficult to cover everything in one session. Between sessions, members will have time to think about what they have learned and to ask questions about anything that is unclear. This type of planning has shown better overall retention and a higher level of members' satisfaction than trying to pack everything into one sitting.

The board chair and the CEO perform specific functions in an orientation program, and the following information should be covered:

### The Board Chair's Role

- **Job description.** The first priority at a new board member orientation is to review the job description with the board chair (see samples in Chapter 1). This review will be much more meaningful if done by the chair and not the CEO because the director is accountable to the chair, not to the CEO. New members can then start off understanding their place in the organization and can relate the rest of the orientation to that perspective. This is also an ideal time for the board chair to review the difference between governance and management information and how the board approaches its proper role.
- **Conflict-of-interest policies.** The board chair should explain the organization's conflict-of-interest policy and disclosure statement. Again, this message will carry more weight coming from the board chair than the CEO. (Appendix 1 and 2 provide samples of these materials.)
- **Attendance and evaluation.** The board chair should cover the expectations of attendance at board meetings and the evaluation processes. The board chair and the new member should share and review a copy of any evaluation forms being used (see appendixes 3 and 4 for samples). When these evaluations are performed, the new member will not be surprised and will understand they are a normal part of the board's routine.

### The CEO's Role

- **Organizational structure.** The CEO should review the hospital's structure aided by a simplified organizational chart. Key positions and their responsibilities should be discussed, and the individuals who fill those positions, along with their backgrounds, should be identified.
- **Review of the healthcare industry.** New board members may not be familiar with issues and trends in the healthcare industry and should be given this information by the CEO, including the following:
    - The latest information on healthcare reform and how it is likely to affect the average hospital will be particularly important
    - Where healthcare fits in the country's overall budget, how much that is per capita, and how that compares with other countries
    - Statistics about the average US hospital should be provided—including numbers of outpatient visits, surgical procedures, and emergency department visits—in comparison with the hospital's actual figures

- The number and types of hospitals; numbers of physicians, nurses, and other healthcare providers in the United States; and the number of people enrolled in managed care plans locally and across the country
- Information about morbidity, mortality, and other quality measures, which will help to put your hospital's statistics into perspective
- Information about the rapidly expanding field of complementary and alternative medicine, including any local impact it has had
- Copies of the most recent healthcare background information and educational materials given to the rest of the board members, so that they will not be lost when such materials are discussed or used in meetings
- **Review of board manuals.** Material with which board members should be familiar and to which they will refer should be compiled and placed in a binder that allows items to be added, deleted, or updated. The CEO should review the following material with new members:
  - The organization's bylaws
  - The organization's mission, vision, goals, objectives, and strategic plan
  - The definition of the board and board member independence
  - A list of board members and resumes for each
  - The functions and limitations of the executive committee, with membership list
  - The functions and responsibilities of other board committees, with membership lists
  - The job description of each board officer
  - The process for removing board members
  - Requirements for annual self-review and collective review of members and the board, including specific assessment tools
  - The organization's market and main challenges
  - The organization's competitors
  - Identification and characteristics of stakeholder groups
  - Responsibilities and processes for monitoring financial and quality-of-care performance, including review of external reporting to governmental and nongovernmental agencies
  - The organization's finances and quality measures
  - An update on any specific projects with which the organization is involved or is contemplating involvement
- **Organizational tour.** Finally, the CEO should take the new board members on a tour of the hospital or, if a system is involved, on a tour of some of the main facilities within the system.

Throughout the orientation process, new members should be made comfortable enough to ask questions or seek clarifications and to request any additional information they deem useful. The goal is to familiarize new board members with the board as quickly and smoothly as possible.

* The author would like to make the following observations:

First, let me say I have been very pro physician my entire career. I have often said I would take a hospital board made up of 100 percent physicians and out-compete anyone if the physicians were the right physicians. My support for physicians began years ago when I was an administrative resident at what is now Northwestern Memorial Hospital in Chicago. For two years I was in the hospital every weekend and holiday as well as evenings and nights as the administrator. The interns and residents were there as the medical staff. I also worked days during the week when the attending physicians were around. This provided considerable interaction with physicians at all levels, and I began to understand how they were trained and how they approached solutions to various problems. After Northwestern, I spent five years in a large teaching hospital in Pennsylvania as an assistant administrator. One of my duties was recruiting interns and residents for the hospital. I was then chosen as the CEO of another hospital in Pennsylvania, and I orchestrated the first merger between an osteopathic and an allopathic hospital in the United States. The views of those two groups of physicians were different in some ways, but similar in others. These experiences formed the foundation for me to relate to physicians in a way that still fosters cooperation.

## References

Bass, K. H. 2008. "Should Physicians Serve on the Board?" *Healthcare Executive* 23 (4): 58–60.

Biggs, E. 2000. "Selecting the Right Physician for Your Board." *Trustee* 53 (9): 22–23.

Collins, J. C. 2001. *Good to Great: Why Some Companies Make the Leap…and Others Don't.* New York: HarperCollins.

Greene, J. 2010. "The Outside Board Member's Perspective." *Trustee.* www.trusteemag.com/trusteemag_app/jsp/articledisplay .jsp?dcrpath=TRUSTEEMAG/Article/data/06JUN2010/1006TRU _coverstory&domain=TRUSTEEMAG.

Trustee Magazine. 2008. "Survey: Boards and Executive Sessions." Hot Topics. *Trustee* 61: 1.

Witt, J. A. 1987. *Building a Better Hospital Board.* Chicago: Health Administration Press.

# CHAPTER FOUR

# How to Work with the CEO

## RELATIONSHIP WITH THE CHIEF EXECUTIVE OFFICER

Ideally, the board and the CEO will work together well and consistently for the benefit of the organization. The relationship can be a complex one, not always developed or maintained easily, but one that can be infinitely rewarding for all concerned, including the hospital.

### The CEO as a Board Member

The CEO works both for and with the board. Pointer and Orlikoff (1999) found more than 80 percent of hospital CEOs are either voting members of their boards or ex officio members without votes. In comparison, almost 80 percent of health-care system CEOs serve as voting members of the board. A study of 90 acute care hospitals in California showed CEO participation as a voting member of the board significantly enhances hospital performance (Molinari, Hendryx, and Goodstein 1997).

As Pointer and Orlikoff (1999) further point out, having the CEO sit on the board as a voting member emphasizes a key characteristic of the unique relationship between the two: The partnership, in addition to the employer–employee aspect, results in better governance. Such a positive result leads to the recommendation that, whenever possible, the CEO also be a voting member of the board. It is in the best interest of the organization.

In such a situation, the CEO knows the board position is an ex officio one, and when she leaves the position, it will be filled by the new CEO. And, of course, the smart CEO would never vote to break a tie among the rest of the board members.

## The Board Is Responsible for One Employee–the CEO

The CEO is the only individual who reports directly to the board and, therefore, is the only one the board evaluates. The board is not responsible for evaluating other employees—including the chief financial officer, chief operating officer, chief nursing officer, and chief medical officer—although the temptation to do so definitely exists for many board members. Although this may be particularly difficult in a smaller community where the board knows so many of these employees, the board must remember that only the CEO is responsible for evaluating all the individuals reporting to him.

Similarly, if a board member perceives a problem with a hospital employee, that member should speak to the CEO about the problem rather than to the employee or the employee's immediate supervisor. The temptation to do otherwise can be strong, but this undermines the authority of the CEO and will usually place both the CEO and the board member in an awkward position.

## CEO Employment Contract

The vast majority of CEOs have employment contracts. In today's turbulent healthcare environment, the decisions required of a CEO are frequently risky and may offend or displease some stakeholders; therefore, an employment contract is essential. The CEO has to be in a position to make decisions, even unpopular ones, in the best interests of the organization.

The American College of Healthcare Executives's (ACHE) Career Resource Center has noted the additional benefits of an employment contract for the healthcare organization and the CEO (Morton 2010):

- An employment contract can help attract and retain competent healthcare leaders by ensuring that there is a mutual understanding of the agreements made between the board and the CEO.
- A contract can also help the board be more objective when reviewing the CEO's performance.
- A contract shows the board's commitment to fair treatment of the CEO if problems develop and allows the board to take a long-term view of the future.

- Additionally, a contract sends a clear signal to various stakeholders that the CEO has the strong support of the board.

For the CEO, a contract

- provides some financial protection,
- clarifies and formalizes the relationship between the CEO and the hospital,
- ensures fair treatment if problems develop, and
- demonstrates the CEO's role as the hospital's main strategist.

A sample CEO employment contract form is shown in Appendix 5.

ACHE also notes the increased use of separation agreements. The intensely challenging environment facing hospitals and their executive leadership portends an increase in involuntary terminations of CEOs. (A sample separation agreement from ACHE is shown in Appendix 6.)

## Evaluation of the CEO

The CEO should be evaluated annually by a committee of the board—usually the executive committee, unless the board has a compensation committee. However, the governance committee may also be a logical choice because it evaluates the full board and individual board members. Individual boards should determine from the start which committee will perform the evaluation so that all lines of communication are clear.

At the beginning of each year the evaluating committee and the CEO should agree on a set of obtainable goals and objectives for the CEO. This is sometimes called a management plan. The management plan serves as a road map for the CEO and an evaluation tool for the committee. Other tools the committee and CEO should use for the evaluation include the following:

- The mission, vision, and goals of the hospital
- A current strategic plan with goals and objectives for the hospital
- The CEO's employment contract and job description
- A job description or the role and responsibilities of the governing board to help provide clarity about the different roles of the board and the CEO
- A shared agreement on the purposes of the CEO evaluation and the evaluation instrument to be used

Having these tools in place will help assure the CEO that her evaluation will be objective and fair. If a crisis occurs, some members of the committee or board may want to deviate from using the management plan as the evaluation tool. How the CEO has handled a crisis may certainly be factored into an evaluation, but the management plan should still be the primary guide. The board or evaluating committee chair must keep the evaluation on track with the agreed-on factors in the management plan and not change horses in midstream or create new rules for evaluating the CEO.

The CEO should be involved in developing the evaluation instrument used by the committee, and each board member should have the opportunity for input to the committee. The evaluation should be conducted in a manner satisfactory to both the committee and the CEO. The outcome of a fair and complete CEO evaluation will benefit both the CEO and the board. The CEO will receive recognition and compensation for his accomplishments, and the board will benefit from seeing the goals of the hospital realized through the CEO's work.

## GOVERNANCE VERSUS MANAGEMENT

Sometimes a fine line exists between management and governance. However, when board members get involved in day-to-day operations, it not only causes problems and requires time-consuming efforts for the CEO and other management personnel, it takes away from the directors' main role of governance. Board members often get involved in operations for the following reasons:

- **A lack of job descriptions.** Having no job description leaves a board member floundering, unsure of what is expected. If a board member clearly sees what the job does and does not entail, there is a better chance she will function according to the job description, in a governance role rather than a managerial one. The importance of board job descriptions is discussed in Chapter 1, and sample job descriptions for board members, the chair, and the vice chair are found in that chapter. A new board member must be given a job description by the board chair, not by the CEO; receiving it from the board chair subtly demonstrates the board's link to governance, not to management.
- **Specialized knowledge.** Board members often have specialized knowledge, and they may feel they should display that knowledge. For example, a certified public accountant on the board may want to be involved in the detailed preparation of financial statements. A general contractor may feel she should be involved in all the hospital's construction projects. Board members are also

usually most comfortable in their areas of expertise, so gravitating to a corresponding area in the hospital's domain may occur unintentionally.

- **Special interests.** Sometimes members have special areas of interest or commitment within the hospital. Perhaps a member's spouse died of a coronary in the hospital, so that board member wants to be involved with issues relating to cardiology services, such as staffing, equipment, a new unit, renovation of the present unit, or cardiology credentialing.
- **Difficulty delegating.** Some board members may be hands-on managers in their regular positions and find it difficult to function at the 30,000-foot level with the rest of the board.
- **Desire to manage during crisis.** Many board members are used to performing many functions in their own businesses, particularly during periods of turbulence or crisis. They may believe getting involved in management activities is helping to save the organization.
- **To fill management voids.** Many times, boards try to fill perceived voids in management. If the hospital has not been able to fill the spot of vice president or another important management position, some board members mistakenly feel they should step in to help with that function.
- **Lack of adequate orientation.** If a good orientation program for new board members does not exist, each will function as he thinks board members should function, without necessarily understanding what is actually expected of him. If all board members have been through a complete and structured orientation, they can help each other to better understand and execute their proper roles.
- **Wrong information.** Sometimes CEOs provide too much management information instead of governance information, giving directors the impression they are being asked to manage. It can be difficult to make sure the board receives only governance information, particularly when some board members want more information and insist on additional reports at meetings. Because few board members will argue with a colleague about the necessity for such reports, the problem is perpetuated. At least every two years the board should critically evaluate the reports and material it receives from management and determine which relate to governance and which to management.

The board chair should work with the CEO to ensure that only governance information is provided to the board. The board's role is to determine where the organization should be headed strategically, and it should not be involved in operations, which is the CEO's job. Although the distinction between governance and management can be fuzzy, just being aware that fuzz exists can help keep the picture clear.

## EXPECTATIONS WHEN WORKING WITH A CEO

Boards must remember they work in partnership with the organization's CEO with the mutual goal of reaching the best decisions and actions for the current and future well-being of the hospital or health system. Appropriate expectations include the following:

- **The CEO works both with and for the board.** As previously noted, most CEOs are members of their boards by virtue of their positions. In this capacity, the CEO works as a strategic partner with the board. However, both will need to remember the board is definitely the employer and the CEO is the employee. As such, the CEO may not be included in every board discussion, such as the CEO evaluation. Today's publicly traded companies are required to have executive sessions without the CEO, even when the CEO is also the chair of the board.
- **The CEO implements the board's policies and directives.** It is the job of the CEO to put into action the plans and directions set by the board. In this role, the CEO functions at 5,000 feet to implement the board's 30,000-foot-level decisions. The CEO deals with hospital personnel, the medical staff, outside contractors, and many others as necessary to ensure the hospital runs smoothly, patients are cared for effectively and efficiently, and the hospital fulfills its mission as set by the board.
- **The board's priorities are the CEO's priorities.** The CEO will provide information to the board about a variety of topics and projects and offer her perspective about the board's proposed course of action; however, once the decision has been made by the board, the CEO becomes the board's hands in getting the work done. The CEO should strive to not get too far ahead of the board or head in a different direction strategically, and she must stay attuned to the board's top priorities for the organization.
- **No surprises.** The CEO should make sure the board does not receive any surprises. The CEO should involve the board early regarding major upcoming decisions so that they can proceed together. Boards do not like to review material and be asked to make major decisions that appear to have already been made. The board should also know both good and bad news before the general public does. It is embarrassing if the media or someone outside the hospital confronts a board member about something that has happened in the hospital if the CEO has not yet informed the board.
- **Involvement in strategic thinking.** An important goal of any board is to ensure the organization is pursuing a winning strategy. The best way to achieve this goal is for the board to be constructively engaged in the hospital's strategic

planning process. If the board is not involved in developing the direction, they may not give their full support for implementing the plan. The board must work closely with the CEO to understand the hospital's needs to ensure the appropriate development, execution, and modification of the organization's strategy.

- **User-friendly board packets.** Before board or committee meetings, board members should not receive thick packets full of management material. Their packets should only contain information related to the decisions they will be making and educational materials to keep them abreast of changes in the healthcare industry. Any CEO who continually does otherwise will lose the support of board members or encourage them to manage rather than govern.

- **Educational opportunities.** The CEO should ensure the board receives relevant industry materials, journals, and educational sessions and attends a well-planned retreat every year. The strongest boards, assisted by their CEOs, will be the ones who know the most about the healthcare industry, what the key issues are, how to function as a board member, and where the hospital should be headed strategically.

- **A program to groom potential board members.** The CEO should work with the governance committee on methods to develop a pool of potential board members. Some hospitals select board members from the hospital's foundation board or allow individuals who are not board members to join board committees.

- **Board member recognition.** The CEO should feature board members in communications about the hospital's newsworthy events, including stories for local media as well as the organization's newsletters and publications. Board members often volunteer many hours each year to the hospital, and this type of attention is an easy way to provide recognition and thanks for their service.

- **Avoiding healthcare jargon.** The board should expect the CEO to refrain from unnecessarily using healthcare jargon. There are numerous abbreviations and acronyms in the healthcare field (see Appendix 7), and members will become familiar with many of them. However, members should not have to sit through meetings without understanding what is being discussed. The smart CEO will cut the use of the jargon as much as possible, and the smart board member will ask questions if something is not understood.

- **Knowing individual board members.** The CEO and board members should develop a mutual understanding and respect for each other's knowledge and strengths. Even in a small community, the CEO should make a point to have lunch at least once a year with each board member. Board members will mention things to the CEO they would never say in a regular board meeting.

- **CEO evaluation.** As mentioned previously, the CEO expects to be evaluated annually to know where improvements need to be made and to have positive achievements recognized.
- **Working with entire board.** In striving to meet expectations, the CEO should work with the entire board, not just the more powerful or vocal members or only the members she gets along with best. Both the CEO and the board will benefit as different members emerge as leaders within the board.

## CEO SUCCESSION PLANNING

According to surveys of directors of public corporations and directors of nonprofit corporations (NACD 2010a; 2010b), CEO succession was an important issue boards should address. Directors of public companies listed it as fifth in importance, behind strategic planning, corporate performance and valuation, financial oversight, and CEO evaluation.

For directors of nonprofit organizations, CEO succession planning ranked 13th out of 25 board issues. The top five issues for these boards were board leadership, ethics and social responsibility, board effectiveness, mission, and strategic planning.

The most effective boards have a formal CEO succession plan. Almost 57 percent of all public companies and 93 percent of the larger public companies have a formal CEO succession plan. Almost 40 percent of nonprofit organizations have a formal CEO succession plan (NACD 2010b).

The succession plans of public companies and nonprofit organizations have three things in common: a process to replace the CEO in the event of an emergency; a development plan for internal candidates; and a process for long-term succession planning (i.e., three to five years before an expected transition).

An ACHE survey (2011) showed CEO turnover in hospitals nationwide was 18 percent annually. Some states had 25 to 32 percent turnover:

- Arkansas, 32 percent
- New Mexico, 32 percent
- Oregon, 31 percent
- South Carolina, 26 percent
- Arizona, 25 percent

ACHE also found the median tenure of CEOs of all general, nonspecialty acute care US hospitals was only 3.6 years. When the CEO leaves, four more senior team members are likely to leave the hospital within one year. The high turnover rate, coupled with a short tenure, should make the board's succession planning function a high priority.

Any healthcare board not planning ahead for the day the CEO leaves is doing the organization a disservice and setting the board up for a difficult transition. One of the most important functions of a board is to ensure the continuation of the organization and to minimize disruption.

The board's role in succession planning breaks down into several components. Although the CEO is the lead in the process, the board should understand it is a joint duty and not one delegated solely to the CEO.

## Committing to the Process

The hospital or health system needs a board and a CEO who believe succession planning is important. The board should make certain the planning is actually being done by bringing it to the attention of the CEO and adding it to his annual performance appraisal objectives. Even the most reluctant CEO will begin planning if he knows a serious discussion will take place annually on the progress made toward this goal.

## Ensuring Smooth Transitions

The board must assign the task of succession planning oversight to a board committee, typically the governance committee. The committee will work closely with the CEO but also needs to have the authority to hire its own outside advisers to help with the process. The CEO will create a succession plan with assistance and advice from the governance committee. The board will then sign off on the plan and, more important, adopt the plan as its own rather than treat it as something the CEO created in a vacuum.

The board makes the ultimate decision on any CEO successor to be named using the plan. Each board will decide how it will interview and observe potential candidates to determine how they think and function as managers and how they might fit with the organization.

A related component of succession planning is planning for transitions on the rest of the executive team. While the board is specifically concerned only with filling the CEO position, it does need to ensure the CEO has a plan for filling vacancies in positions such as the chief financial officer, the chief operating officer, the medical director, or the director of nursing. Having a sound plan for making smooth transitions in all top leadership positions will certainly help the hospital move forward with its mission, vision, and goals without pause.

---

**Challenges of Succession Planning**

Succession planning is not necessarily easy, and boards may face certain problems when developing or working with a CEO succession plan:

- *Assumptions change quickly.* Succession plans make assumptions, and in a fast-changing environment, assumptions can change quickly. The hospital that was a freestanding facility last month may decide this month to join a system or to create a system on its own. A main internal candidate may thus need to be passed over as CEO-designate as part of a bargaining position or in deference to perceived equity with the other entity.
- *Boards change.* A change in board leadership may mean a change in how a succession plan will be implemented. A new board chair may look at any internal candidates differently or be unwilling to be held to the plan of the previous chair. This is one reason promises made must be carefully thought through. Although promises of this nature tend not to be in writing, boards should avoid making or breaking them.
- *The internal candidate is unable to assume the position.* The heir apparent may not be ready or able to succeed the CEO. This can come about through failure on the successor's part or because designating a formal replacement may be the equivalent of placing a target on that person's back. In the latter situation, issues surrounding the departing CEO may be transferred to the heir apparent, who then becomes the target for ill will directed at the departing or departed CEO. This may create an untenable situation for both the board and the successor, doing the hospital a great disservice.
- *Other capable employees may leave.* Designating an heir apparent may cause the departure of others in the organization who might be well qualified by the time the CEO steps aside. Because of this, some organizations might indicate to several potential candidates they are being considered as CEO replacements. The question then becomes whether the potential replacements can continue to support each other as team members in an environment where only one will eventually be selected.

---

## Keeping Promises

Once the succession planning process is completed, the board should make sure any promises it has made are communicated to succeeding board leadership and those promises are kept. In general, however, the board should limit itself to as few promises as possible; this leaves succeeding boards with the flexibility required in these rapidly changing times.

## Appointing an Acting CEO

If the board has tried succession planning but has had little success in creating a satisfactory plan, or if the hospital needs a new CEO before a plan has been completed, a few alternatives are available to provide time until a new CEO can be named. Many healthcare organizations have found it necessary to go outside the organization to look for the new CEO. This may be because internal candidates are not deemed adequate, a change in direction or philosophy is called for, or no internal candidate wants the job. Sometimes an outside search is conducted even when an excellent candidate exists internally; this is usually done when the board wants to make sure the new CEO is the best available at the time. The outside search may or may not validate the selection of the internal candidate.

To minimize the disruption created when a CEO departs unexpectedly, an internal individual can be designated as the acting CEO. Typically, the acting CEO is the leading candidate for the job. Sometimes, however, the board decides to bring in an interim leader whose sole job is to hold things together until a new CEO is appointed. With someone in the CEO's chair, decisions can be made allowing the hospital to continue moving forward while the search continues.

CEO succession planning is definitely an important function a board must address. The board should openly talk about succession planning and consider some of the following questions:

1. What is the best way for the board to ensure a smooth succession?
2. How should the management development and succession process be handled?
3. How should the board work with the present CEO during the succession process?
4. What makes for a strong CEO candidate?
5. What role should an executive search firm play?
6. When should outside candidates be considered?
7. How much competition should be encouraged among potential CEO candidates?
8. Should the former CEO play any role after she is succeeded?
9. How many years before an expected CEO transition should the board begin the succession planning process?
10. How should the board interact with internal candidates?
11. What can the board do to successfully involve all board members in the succession planning process?

If the board openly addresses the need for a plan that asks these questions, it is well on its way to developing an effective succession process. The real secret of successful hiring and firing of CEOs is having a good succession process which reduces the board's risk of hiring the wrong CEO or having to fire anyone.

## References

American College of Healthcare Executives (ACHE). 2011. "Annual CEO Turnover by State." *Modern Healthcare* 40: 32.

Molinari, C., M. Hendryx, and J. Goodstein. 1997. "The Effects of CEO-Board Relations on Hospital Performance." *Health Care Management Review* 22 (3): 7–15.

Morton, R. L. 2010. *Employment Contracts for Healthcare Executives,* 5th ed. Chicago: Health Administration Press.

National Association of Corporate Directors (NACD). 2010a "2009–2010 NACD Public Company Governance Survey." Washington, DC: National Association of Corporate Directors.

———. 2010b. "2009 NACD Nonprofit Governance Survey." Washington, DC: National Association of Corporate Directors.

Pointer, D. D., and J. E. Orlikoff. 1999. *Board Work: Governing Health Care Organizations.* San Francisco: Jossey-Bass.

Tyler, J. L., and E. L. Biggs. 2001. *Practical Governance.* Chicago: Health Administration Press.

# CHAPTER FIVE

# How to Ensure Quality Care

## MONITORING QUALITY OF HEALTHCARE

*Michael Pugh, president, Verisma Systems, Inc., Pueblo, Colorado*

### Board Responsibility for Quality and Performance

"Isn't that what the doctors and nurses are supposed to be doing?" is a common first thought when new hospital board members are told that patient safety and the quality of care are ultimately the board's legal responsibility. While physicians and nurses are critical to the quality process, and having well-trained and appropriately credentialed professionals on the staff is important, considerably more is required for boards to carry out their legal and fiduciary responsibilities for quality. Boards must have a broad view and understanding of quality to ensure that patient care is safe, effective, and reliable.

For many years, graduate programs in healthcare administration taught a model of hospital organization using the metaphor of a three-legged stool, with the administration, the board, and the medical staff as the legs of the stool supporting a platform for patient care delivery. The board was responsible for fundraising and gathering community input, the administration for staffing and operating the hospital, and the medical staff for bringing patients to the hospital and providing care. Board members assumed the quality was high if the hospital had well-trained doctors, state-of-the art technology and facilities, low staff turnover, satisfied patients, and generally clean reports from auditors, regulators, and accreditation agencies. While these proxies for describing good quality are important and contribute to high-quality patient care and experiences, simply equating quality to facilities, doctors, or reputation does not fulfill the board's responsibility for ensuring that patient care is safe and every patient gets exactly the right care, every time.

For more than 200 years, the "three-legged stool" description, sometimes called the Franklin Model (based on the hospital concept used by Benjamin Franklin when he founded The Pennsylvania Hospital in the late 1700s), paralleled the basic legal responsibilities of doctors and hospitals. But beginning in the 1960s a series of legal decisions, most notably *Darling v. Charleston Community Memorial Hospital* (211 N.E.2d 253,1965), established the hospital board was ultimately responsible for the outcomes of patient care.

**Credentialing.** During the 1970s and 1980s, the primary tool for ensuring quality was the medical staff appointment and reappointment process. Sometimes referred to as credentialing, this process established the level of care and procedures that individual physicians were allowed to perform based on their training and experience. Physicians would apply for membership to the medical staff, and the hospital board would rely on a recommendation from the existing medical staff to allow physicians to admit patients to the hospital. The underlying hospital quality theory in the 1970s and 1980s: Keep the "bad" physicians off the medical staff.

**Peer review.** As an extension of the credentialing process, hospitals and medical staffs established peer review and other mechanisms to investigate and monitor individual physician performance; these efforts focused on the mistakes or errors a physician might have made in the care of patients. Recommendations to the governing board for corrective action might range from no action to relatively benign corrective actions, such as a letter to reprimand a physician or requirements for additional training. In some cases, recommendations might involve limiting privileges to perform certain procedures, or in extreme cases, terminating all care privileges and expulsion from the medical staff. The more punitive the potential board action, the greater the risk the board, hospital, or physicians involved in the peer review might be sued for violating the due process standards in the medical staff bylaws, which are meant to ensure fairness and impartiality in the review process.

In most states, the deliberations and investigations surrounding peer review have some measure of confidentiality and protection from legal discovery. But that is cold comfort for most physicians asked to be involved in the process. While the intent of peer review is good, the process is sometimes difficult and potentially flawed. Fear of lawsuits, potential conflicts of interest, variations in the professional knowledge of the reviewers, social relationships, closed sessions without nurses or others with a perspective present, and an unspoken but inherent reluctance among physicians to criticize their colleagues tend to diminish the potential impact and benefit of peer review on overall quality. Occasionally, suggestions do come out of the peer review process that might improve the care for all patients, but such suggestions are a byproduct of the process and not the focus of the effort.

**Quality assurance.** In the 1970s and 1980s, a quality control process known as quality assurance (QA) also emerged. In the QA process, patient charts were pulled after the patient was discharged and reviewed for the appropriateness and quality of care. The charts selected for review might have been pulled because of a patient complaint or known problem with the care, were sometimes selected for a routine review of specific types of admissions or might have been a random selection of charts. In some hospitals, but not all, efforts were made to ensure that every physician on the active medical staff had at least a few charts reviewed each year. Generally, the criteria for chart selection was determined by a committee of the medical staff and the charts were prescreened by a registered nurse (RN) employed by the hospital looking for specific issues, usually related to compliance with Medicare and Medicaid regulations. If the nurse noted a problem or gap in care, the chart was referred to a physician reviewer. If the physician reviewer felt the physician care was inadequate, the chart might be referred to a peer review committee that would investigate further. If the care by the hospital staff was poor or something bad had happened such as a fall, but it was not a physician mistake, the chart might be sent to risk management or referred to someone in management. Because Medicare and Medicaid reimbursement was often at stake, efforts were usually focused on improving documentation and payment issues. While some useful information was occasionally gleaned, leading to overall improvements in care, for the most part QA used the same quality theory as peer review: Find and eliminate the bad apples.

However, removing the bad apple from the barrel does nothing to improve the quality of the rest of the apples in the barrel. Credentialing, peer review, and QA remain important and necessary, but these efforts generally do not result in quality improvement for all patients, and they are not processes that completely fulfill the board's ultimate responsibility for quality care.

## A Different View of Hospital Quality

In the late 1980s, the theories and methods to improve quality and reduce manu-facturing defects began to be understood and adapted in healthcare. The key breakthrough in thinking about quality in healthcare was the realization that poor quality outcomes were most often the result of system or process failure rather than individual physician or staff failure or just bad luck. Quality became a process problem, not a people problem. Physicians are a critical part of the process, but not the entire care process—a lot of other people are involved.

As an example, surgeons are sometimes compared or judged by their surgical-site infection rate. However, the surgeon rarely cleans the equipment, cleans the operating room, maintains the ventilation system, shaves the patient, prepares the surgical site, starts the prescribed antibiotic in the effective window prior to surgery, or controls the glycogen levels of the patient during surgery. How well these tasks are carried out is known to decrease the probability of a surgical site infection by as much as 90 percent, but they are out of the effective control or direct influence of the surgeon. So while surgical technique and maintaining a sterile field during sur-gery are clearly important, are surgical site infections a doctor problem or a hospital system problem? The answer is likely some unknown and unknowable combina-tion. However, across the country, the rigorous adherence to a set of simple basic operating room tasks—such as hand washing, proper preparation of the surgical site, and the timely administration of antibiotics—has been shown to dramatically reduce the overall incidence of surgical-site infections.

Dr. Paul Batalden, a cofounder and the first chair of the board of the Institute for Healthcare Improvement (IHI), said it best: "Every system is perfectly designed to produce the results it gets" (McInnis 2006). Batalden's observation is grounded in statistical process control theory, which postulates that any stable process produces variation in outputs—some will be good and some will be bad. The required management action is not to chase the bad results but to change the process so it consistently produces the desired results. While perfectly logical, the idea that processes, rather than doctors, are the root of many of the poor outcomes in healthcare has been slow to take root.

System and process thinking got a major boost in 2000 when the government-sponsored Institute of Medicine (IOM) published *To Err Is Human* and in 2002 followed up with a second report, *Crossing the Quality Chasm*. The first report highlighted how error and poor quality were rampant in healthcare and reported that between 98,000 and 140,000 patients died unnecessarily each year in US hospitals, making hospital deaths the eighth leading cause of death, ahead of motor vehicle fatalities. As expected, there were fierce attacks on the report and challenges to the estimated number of preventable deaths and the ideas presented. However, since the original publication, other studies and estimates suggest the IOM understated the enormity of the problem.

The second report advocated healthcare redesign along the principles of safe, effective, efficient, patient-centered, cost-efficient, and equitable care for all. While initially controversial, the IOM reports served as a wake-up call for hospitals to begin thinking about quality and patient outcomes much differently. In the decade since the IOM reports, awareness has developed that many of the things we used to consider complications in the treatment of patients are actually avoidable patient-harm events. Potentially fatal hospital-acquired conditions—such as ventilator-associated pneumonia, sepsis, infections associated with venous catheters, and medication errors—can effectively be eliminated by strict adherence to simple care and procedure protocols.

Dr. Donald Berwick (2003), the founder and former president of IHI and now administrator of the Centers for Medicare & Medicaid Services (CMS), has said when you strip everything else away, what patients are really saying is

1. Don't hurt me.
2. Help me.
3. Be nice to me.

These three patient-centered elements, in the order of priority listed, redefine how we think about quality in healthcare. "First, do no harm" is part of the Hippocratic Oath all physicians take upon graduation—an old idea. But for healthcare organizations, "Don't hurt me" is a relatively new foundation to organizational quality improvement efforts. Unfortunately, as reported by the IOM, patient harm is widespread and insidious. In 2006, IHI launched its 5 Million Lives Campaign, aimed at encouraging hospitals to take steps to significantly reduce harm to patients. As part of that campaign, IHI (2006) adopted and published a broad and inclusive definition of patient harm:

Unintended physical injury resulting from or contributed to by medical care (including the absence of indicated medical treatment) that requires additional monitoring, treatment or hospitalization, or that results in death. Such injury is considered harm whether or not it is considered preventable, resulted from a medical error, or occurred within a hospital.

Hospitals and other healthcare organizations typically keep track of the number of falls, infections, medication errors, wrong-site surgeries, delayed treatments, bed sores, procedural mishaps, and other potential patient-harm events. However, this information may be gathered by different people for disparate purposes and is rarely compiled on an organization-wide basis. Reports on falls are separate from reports on infections, which are separate from reports on medication errors and so on. To further muddy the waters, harm is often reported as a rate per 1,000 patient days or some other denominator that tends to diminish the impact of the data. Board members, management, and medical staff leadership are routinely shocked the first time the aggregate actual number of harm events is presented—almost always much higher than expected. Boards need to ask to see the actual number of harm events and then set aggressive targets for reduction.

The second plea, "Help me," is typically why most individuals choose healthcare as a career—they want to help other people. "Help me" does not mean "cure me." Most patients are realistic in their expectations of what medicine can and cannot do. What they really want is for the healthcare system to reliably deliver everything that is known to help. Hospitals face two problems in meeting this need. The first is defining what is known to help. Numerous studies over the past decade have shown tremendous geographic variation in the treatment for almost all medical conditions and wide disparities in healthcare costs (Dartmouth 2011). The second problem is, after defining what is known to help based on clinical evidence, building the processes and systems to ensure that the "right care" is always delivered.

The IOM has estimated 30 percent of what is spent on healthcare in the United States adds no clinical value. Other studies suggest only about 50 percent of all care delivered is actually evidence-based, meaning there is hard, replicable science linking the treatment and the outcome.

The practical application of evidence-based medicine had its roots in an obstetrics malpractice insurance crisis in the late 1970s and early 1980s. In response, the American College of Obstetrics and Gynecology began publishing guidelines to help practicing physicians who agreed to practice according to the guidelines to obtain or maintain malpractice insurance. Next, in 2004, Medicare began measuring the quality of care in hospitals with a set of core measures that tracked whether the common evidence-based clinical treatment elements were delivered for the conditions of heart attack, pneumonia, congestive heart failure, and stroke.

Medicare's action helped hospitals and physicians begin to think differently about the use of protocols and standardized care plans and spurred the concept of the "right care"—delivering evidence-based care every time for every patient.

Many hospitals have fallen into the trap of looking at the percentage of time individual care elements were delivered rather than how often patients receive all of the required care elements. If a patient qualifies for six elements in an evidence-based care plan, but the hospital only delivers four, did the patient get the right care? Numerous studies have shown hospitals that can reliably deliver all of the care according to the evidence have lower mortality and complication rates (Mukherjee et al. 2004; Eagle et al. 2005).

The third patient desire—"Be nice to me"—is reflected in patient satisfaction data. During the 1990s, almost all hospitals began focusing on patient satisfaction, conducting surveys and adapting service techniques from other industries to improve the patient experience. In 2009, Medicare began publishing comparative patient satisfaction statistics for all hospitals, available on the CMS website. Service quality and amenities are important, but a smiling nurse and valet parking will not likely offset the experience from a hospital-acquired infection, a wrong-site surgery, or a medication error resulting in harm.

## Board Strategies for Measuring and Improving Quality

The board is ultimately responsible for everything happening in the hospital, including reducing harm and ensuring care is delivered appropriately and according to the evidence. There are four common challenges with which boards and new board members may struggle:

1. **Getting comfortable with the board's responsibility for the care and safety of patients.** Getting comfortable requires boards to have good processes in place for credentialing, discussing difficult issues, and resolving conflicts. There is no ambiguity about a board's legal responsibility for care and outcomes. But it takes a strong management and medical staff team and good board relations to be transparent and openly discuss patient harm and poor quality outcomes—topics that in most hospital environments have not traditionally engendered trust between the board, management, and physician leadership. As the nursing staff plays such an important role in the delivery of quality patient care on a 24-hour-a-day, 7-day-a-week basis, the board must be willing to appropriately involve nursing leadership in these discussions as well. Most CEOs did not get to be the CEO by delivering bad news. Boards have a responsibility to create a board meeting environment in which difficult issues can be discussed without fear of punishment.

The way to begin to build the right board environment is by asking inquiry questions, not attack questions. Board members should feel comfortable asking governance questions about quality, such as

- How many patients were harmed last month?
- How does that compare to the previous six months?
- Are we trending downward?
- What are the plans for the next wave of efforts to reduce patient falls, medication errors, hospital-acquired infections?
- What percentage of the care delivered in our cardiac program was "right care"?

These questions are no different from the types of questions the finance committee asks about financial issues: Where are we, are we getting better, what is your strategy for improvement?

2. **Setting the right expectations for the organization's leadership and medical and nursing staffs.** Setting the right quality expectations and having a good process to monitor progress are the two most important things a board can do in exercising its responsibility for quality patient care and preventing harm. Recent studies have shown that better outcomes are associated with hospitals in which:

- The board spends more than 25 percent of its time on quality issues.
- The board receives a formal quality performance measurement report.
- There is a high level of interaction between the board and the medical staff on quality strategy.
- The senior executives' compensation is based in part on quality improvement (QI) performance.
- The CEO is identified as the person with the greatest impact on QI, especially when so identified by the QI executive (usually a physician on the hospital payroll who has responsibility for implementing QI programs).

The key is setting the right governance aims. Hospital boards should set aggressive aims seeking to dramatically reduce levels of harm to patients. External comparative data are not necessary and, in fact, counterproductive when it comes to harm—there is no appropriate level of harm, especially if you are the patient. All that is required is a simple monthly or quarterly count of the number of patients who experienced harm. Some organizations have developed composite indicators that measure not only patient harm but also the number of serious safety events whether the patient was harmed or not, on the theory that the focus should be on preventing any event that could lead to harm.

The board must also set "what by when" targets (e.g., reduce all harm events by 50 percent by December 2013), which will create the expectation that significant process change is required to reach the targets, not an incremental or marginal approach to improvement.

3. **Getting useful information and monitoring performance.** The board should also focus on what is important—high-level outcomes rather than detail. For far too long, hospital boards have suffered from an excess of data and a dearth of information from quality reports. Instead, the board should focus its review and discussion on a few high-level outcome measures that can be presented in a fairly simple scorecard or report format. The scorecard should include measures and targets for the following:

- Hospital mortality tracked over time (run chart)
- Number of patient safety and harm events, tracked over time
- Unplanned hospital readmission rate
- Percentage of time care is provided according to the evidence (right care)
- Patient satisfaction

Measures on the board's quality scorecard should be limited to the most important areas to provide governance and not management oversight. The organization's quality and operating strategies should be linked and should drive the measures in the desired direction.

In some organizations, boards may need to add a few other measures specific to the mission of the organization or challenges faced by the organization. Those types of measures might include the following:

- A measure that represents access or waiting time in clinics or emergency facilities
- A measure representing culture or staff satisfaction
- A measure representing cost efficiency or value
- A measure representing equity in care across demographics

The most effective boards have active quality committees that begin their meetings with a brief story of a patient experience, effectively putting a face on the data. The committee typically reviews the board's quality aims and targets and progress toward achieving those quality aims. It also reviews the execution and quality improvement plans the medical staff and management propose for the next month or quarter. Further, the committee should review sentinel events and reports of harm and review regulatory dashboards for compliance exceptions; it may also periodically receive reports from risk management. Finally, the committee should consider any policy change recommendations which may require full board approval. Some boards use the quality committee to review medical staff credentialing recommendations prior to a vote by the full board. The chair of the quality committee, not the management team, should make the committee report to the full board.

Dr. James Reinertsen (2011), a senior fellow at IHI, advocates including patients on the quality committee of the board. Board members may occasionally be patients, but their experiences, because of their access and status in the organization, often do not represent the experiences of other patients. More importantly, a board member's fiduciary duty is to the organization. Patients in the boardroom tend to reduce self-serving conversations and add a perspective no one else in the room is free to deliver.

4. **Creating accountability for quality results.** The final challenge is to create accountability for quality results. Many hospitals are beginning to tie CEO and senior leader compensation to the achievement of strategic and quality goals. When structured correctly, compensation can align management actions with the board's goals and expectations. Organization-wide accountability is also created through transparency of aims, targets, and progress. Boards that spend as much time discussing quality issues at their meetings as they do financial and operating issues send a clear message to the organization, which can drive cultural change and foster accountability.

## The Business Case for Quality

Whether or not there is a financial case supporting a specific improvement strategy, there is always a business case for improving quality in healthcare. Poor quality represents waste in the hospital and healthcare system. Across the country, hospitals are learning that when they eliminate or dramatically reduce ventilator-associated pneumonias, central line infections, medication errors, and patient falls, operating costs go down, not up. Quality in healthcare does cost less when waste in the form of patient harm is reduced.

In 2008, Medicare began eliminating payment when any "never events" occur and reducing payment for complications that occur in the hospital. Depending on state regulations the event may be reportable to a public agency or to The Joint Commission.

**Never-Event CMS Regulatory Categories**

1. Air embolisms
2. Mediastinitis—surgical site infection after coronary artery bypass graft
3. Catheter-associated urinary tract infections
4. Vascular catheter-associated infections
5. Blood incompatibility
6. Objects left in the patient during surgery
7. Falls, trauma
8. Pressure ulcers
9. Poorly controlled blood sugar
10. Infections after elective orthopedic and bariatric surgery
11. Deep vein thrombosis or pulmonary embolisms following total hip and knee replacement

Other payers have followed with even more restrictive policies. Under the 2009 healthcare reform legislation, the pressures ratchet up on hospitals with increasing payment reductions if the hospital has a higher-than-expected rate of readmissions, and expands those quality penalties to the Medicaid program. Not many carrots, but lots of sticks. Healthcare reform also envisions value purchasing—forcing hospitals to reduce costs to show greater value. Improving quality and reducing harm may be the most powerful value strategy on the board's strategy scorecard.

*The Joint Commission is unique in its predominance and influence as an accrediting body for healthcare organizations. Members of governing boards should determine if the features described in the following section would benefit their organization. If so, accreditation should be sought.*

*Errol L. Biggs*

## THE JOINT COMMISSION
*Cathy Barry-Ipema, chief communications officer, The Joint Commission*

Founded in 1951, The Joint Commission is the nation's leading evaluator of healthcare quality and safety; eight out of ten hospitals nationwide are voluntarily accredited by The Joint Commission.

The Joint Commission is an independent, not-for-profit organization that inspires healthcare organizations to excel in providing effective care of the highest quality and safety. The Joint Commission sets the standards by which healthcare quality and safety are measured in the United States and around the world. It is

## The Board and Healthcare Quality

New board members generally face a steep learning curve for ensuring quality in healthcare. But that curve can be flattened if they keep a few things in mind and in perspective:

1.  Ultimately the board is legally responsible for the quality of care and service provided.

2.  Medical staff credentialing and peer review are important but alone are insufficient to ensure good quality. Having good doctors does not automatically equate to decreased harm and better outcomes.

3.  Every system is perfectly designed to produce the results it gets. Poor quality and patient harm are generally the results of flawed systems and processes.

4.  Patients have three requirements: Don't hurt me, help me, and be nice to me. Quality in healthcare is about delivering on all three.

5.  The board should track a few key quality metrics and set aggressive targets to set expectations and create organizational and strategic focus.

6.  The quality committee of the board is the primary mechanism for monitoring quality performance and improvement efforts.

7.  There is a strong business case for improving quality and reducing harm.

8.  Ask lots of questions. The only dumb question is the one not asked.

governed by a 29-member board that includes physicians, administrators, nurses, employers, ethicists, and consumers, and it evaluates more than 19,000 healthcare organizations. These include hospitals, nursing homes, home care agencies, behavioral healthcare organizations, outpatient clinics, laboratories, office-based surgery practices, and critical access hospitals.

To earn and maintain accreditation, organizations must have an extensive onsite review by a team of healthcare professionals (surveyors) at least once every three years. This rigorous review evaluates an organization's performance in areas that directly affect patient care. Accreditation may then be awarded based on how well the organization has met Joint Commission standards.

The standards cover important areas such as medication management, infection prevention and control, patient safety, patient care, staff qualifications, patient rights, leadership, and environment of care. The Joint Commission has made significant changes to the accreditation process, progressively sharpening the focus of the process on the operational systems most critical to the safety and quality of patient care. Critical elements of Joint Commission accreditation are its standards, performance measures, the periodic performance review process, and an unannounced onsite survey (which includes the use of data from multiple sources to help guide the survey) that includes tracking an individual's patient care experiences.

Although The Joint Commission accreditation process is complex, many factors encourage healthcare facilities to seek this status:

1. The Joint Commission standards are focused on one goal: raising, to the highest possible level, the safety and quality of care provided to the public. Joint Commission standards include state-of-the-art performance improvement concepts to help organizations continually improve their quality and safety of care.

2. Accreditation highlights an organization's dedication to providing safe and high-quality care to the community it serves. Achieving accreditation makes a strong statement to the community about an organization's commitment to provide the highest-quality services.

3. The survey process is designed to be educational and supportive. The Joint Commission surveyors are experienced healthcare professionals trained to provide a rigorous evaluation and expert observations during the survey. In addition to evaluating current practices at the organization being surveyed, they focus on improving systems and processes and sharing leading practices. Recommendations for improvement are provided.

4. The Joint Commission offers many educational seminars and publications about performance improvement and other standards-related topics. In addition, account executives and members of The Joint Commission's Standards Interpretation Group can provide immediate assistance and suggestions on standards interpretation and compliance and the survey process.

5. Accreditation can help lessen the burden imposed by duplicative federal and state regulatory agency surveys. Some accredited healthcare organizations may qualify for Medicare and Medicaid certification without undergoing a separate government survey.

6. Several states recognize Joint Commission accreditation as fulfilling some or all of the state's hospital licensing requirements.

7. Increasingly, accreditation is becoming a prerequisite to eligibility for insurance reimbursement, for participation in managed care plans, and for bidding on contracts.

8. By enhancing risk-management efforts, accreditation may improve access to and reduce the cost of liability insurance coverage.

9. Case managers and other healthcare professionals frequently use accreditation as a benchmark of quality when placing individuals. Staff, including

physicians and nurses, may also consider Joint Commission status of the organization before deciding to affiliate with it.

10. Lenders may require accreditation as a condition of financing, assuming that accredited organizations may be more capable of paying debt than unaccredited ones.

Although all 10 of these factors will not apply to every healthcare organization, their merits should be considered by management and the board of directors when determining whether to seek Joint Commission accreditation. It is certainly one way in which healthcare organizations can actively demonstrate their commitment to quality and safe patient care.


## DRIVING ACCOUNTABILITY FOR IMPROVED QUALITY AND OUTCOMES IN YOUR COMMUNITY: BUSINESS COALITIONS ON HEALTH

*Donna Marshall, executive director, Colorado Business Group on Health*

More than 50 locations in the United States have a business coalition on health that is affiliated with the National Business Coalition on Health and designed to improve value and quality in healthcare for members and the larger community. In other words, they have been formed to reduce the trend in rising healthcare costs and to increase healthcare quality for the employees of their member companies. Both hospital board members and business coalition members are often local community business leaders and as such should collaborate to deliver a shared vision of accountable and affordable healthcare.

Most coalitions are 501(c)(3) or 501(c)(6) not-for-profit entities; about 5 percent are for profit.

Coalitions that belong to the National Business Coalition on Health have 7,000 employer members that boast a collective population of 10.3 million employees and 25 million covered lives throughout the country.

At least two coalitions number more than 1 million employees each: the Pacific Business Group on Health and the Washington Business Group on Health (which is independent from the National Business Coalition on Health). Many business coalitions thrive in midsized markets of about 500,000 people, where coalitions can effectively forge relationships with larger employers and interact with a less complex medical marketplace. Some examples include The Alliance of Madison, Wisconsin, and Nevada Health Care Coalition of Reno, Nevada (see Exhibit 5.1 for names of states where current business coalitions are located).

**Exhibit 5.1: Locations of Business Coalitions That Belong to the National Business Coalition on Health**

**Arkansas**
Employers' Health Coalition

**California**
Pacific Business Group on Health

**Colorado**
Colorado Business Group on Health

**Florida**
Florida Health Care Coalition

**Georgia**
Savannah Business Group on Health

**Hawaii**
Hawaii Business Health Council

**Illinois**
Employers' Coalition on Health
Heartland Healthcare Coalition
Midwest Business Group on Health
Tri-State Health Care Coalition

**Indiana**
Indiana Employers Quality Health Alliance
Tri-State Business Group on Health

**Kansas**
Wichita Business Coalition on Health Care

**Louisiana**
Louisiana Health Care Alliance

**Maine**
Maine Health Management Coalition

**Maryland**
MidAtlantic Business Group on Health

**Michigan**
Michigan Purchasers Health Alliance

**Minnesota**
Buyers Health Care Action Group
Labor/Management Health Care Coalition of the Upper Midwest

**Missouri**
Mid-America Coalition on Health Care
St. Louis Area Business Health Coalition

**Montana**
Montana Association of Health Care Purchasers

**Nevada**
Health Services Coalition
Nevada Health Care Coalition

**New Jersey**
New Jersey Health Care Quality Institute

**New York**
New York Business Group on Health
Niagara Health Quality Coalition

**North Carolina**
Piedmont Health Coalition, Inc.
Western North Carolina Health Coalition

**Ohio**
Employers Health Purchasing Corporation of Ohio
FrontPath Health Coalition
Health Action Council Ohio

**Oregon**
Oregon Coalition of Health Care Purchasers

**Pennsylvania**
Employers Health Coalition of Pennsylvania, Inc.
Lancaster County Business Group on Health
Lehigh Valley Business Coalition on Health Care
Pittsburgh Business Group on Health

**Rhode Island**
Rhode Island Business Group on Health

**South Carolina**
South Carolina Business Coalition on Health

**Tennessee**
Healthcare 21 Business Coalition
Memphis Business Group on Health

*(continued)*

**Exhibit 5.1** *(continued)*

**Texas**
    Dallas/Fort Worth Business Group on
      Health
    Houston Business Group on Health
    Texas Business Group on Health
**Virginia**
    Virginia Business Coalition on Health
**Washington**
    Puget Sound Health Alliance

**Wisconsin**
    The Alliance
    Business Health Care Group
    Fond Du Lac Area Businesses on
      Health
    Greater Milwaukee Business
      Foundation on Health, Inc.
    WisconsinRx and National
      CooperativeRx
**Wyoming**
    Wyoming Business Coalition on Health

SOURCE: NCBH (2009).

## Business Coalition Goals

Wisely purchasing healthcare benefits for an employee population is a difficult task. Most business coalitions are formed when a small number of dedicated employers rally around the concept of value-based purchasing. Value-based purchasing is different from typical healthcare purchasing: both cost and quality are incorporated into the assessment, selection, and ongoing monitoring of healthcare services. Key features of coalition activities include

- Value-based purchasing
- Acquisition of healthcare utilization and cost data
- Standardization of performance measures
- Creation of health plan and hospital performance reports
- Education of coalition members and the greater community
- Education of employees and other citizens
- Legislative advocacy and monitoring

Purchasers join together as they realize the benefits of using a coalition to implement value-based purchasing. They use their combined strengths to create negotiating leverage in the marketplace. They share information and resources to create standardized requests for proposals, performance standards, and healthcare data collecting and reporting.

One aspect of value-based purchasing translates into group purchasing arrangements for the majority of coalitions. Coalition members may join to purchase health plans, preferred provider networks, pharmacy benefit management services, or other healthcare services such as dental and vision plans. Other coalitions have built local or regional preferred provider networks, and their member companies enjoy coalition-negotiated discounts. Business coalition members are discussing the possible re-emergence of direct contracting and narrow provider networks to enhance their opportunity for more cost-effective and higher-quality outcomes. Even when a coalition is not purchasing, these kinds of discussions between businesses and hospitals will influence the local healthcare marketplace.

Some business coalitions have embraced innovations for improving quality, financing, and delivery systems of healthcare in their markets. Thirty-four coalitions support the Leapfrog Group in their regions, and six have adopted programs to reward top-performing physicians in the national Bridges to Excellence initiative. Business coalitions have formed or are participating in data initiatives, such as all payer claims databases or regional health information organizations, medical home initiatives, and accountable care collaboratives.

## Business Coalition Perspective and Recent Studies

Mission statements of nearly all business coalitions address quality of healthcare. Coalition members acknowledge the many opportunities and obligations members have to improve the structure, financing, and accountability of the healthcare marketplace.

In today's increasingly competitive market, healthcare purchasers are looking beyond the direct cost of premiums and looking instead at the combined costs of direct spending and lost productivity and absenteeism in the worksite due to the poor health of employees. Research conducted by the Dartmouth Institute of Health Policy and Clinical Practice documents variations in healthcare spending and utilization that, for unexplained reasons, may not have directly related to better outcomes for patients: numbers of physician and specialist visits, number and frequency of tests, average length of stay in hospitals, and morbidity and mortality rates for common inpatient procedures. At the same time, common cost-effective and medically endorsed interventions (such as administration of aspirin in the emergency department for patients with a suspected heart attack or prevention of deep vein thrombosis after common surgical procedures) are not always routinely performed. More expensive healthcare and poor clinical outcomes for employees are a poor investment from a purchaser's view.

A widely cited study, published by the Midwest Business Group on Health in collaboration with the Juran Institute and The Sevryn Group, Inc. (2003), asserts the cost of poor-quality care amounts to about 30 percent of healthcare expenditures. This study uses the paradigm of "overuse, underuse, and misuse" to document activities that do not improve the value equation in healthcare. The next step is to determine how employers can define and differentiate high-quality healthcare when they decide how to spend their healthcare dollars. The Midwest Business Group on Health report is a road map for changing purchasing behavior.

*To Err Is Human* (IOM 2000) asserts that patient safety is one of the most important issues confronting the healthcare system. Its estimate that between 44,000 and 98,000 people die in hospitals each year due to errors presents a toll in both human and financial terms that is indefensible. The focus now is to reform the current system in three fundamental ways:

1. Engendering a culture of safety, instead of the current blame-and-shame paradigm;
2. Acknowledging most errors are system errors because common processes have not been engineered to ensure safety; and
3. Confronting the appalling lack of information on quality outcomes and reduction of waste.

## Business Coalitions in Action: The Leapfrog Group

An outgrowth of the report was the creation of the Leapfrog Group, initiated in 2000 by a group of *Fortune* 100 companies to demand higher levels of performance accountability by hospitals and ultimately change payment systems to reward higher quality. Business leaders from The Business Roundtable called together academic and medical experts to advocate for a small number of improvements, called the *three leaps*, to dramatically improve safety in the nation's hospitals. The three leaps were also selected because their adoption enhances structural changes within the industry.

1. Leap one: Implement a computerized pharmacy order-entry system for all inpatient medication ordering by physicians.
2. Leap two: Use specially trained hospitalists (intensivists) to staff intensive care units.
3. Leap three: Bring focus for consumers and purchasers to select institutions meeting certain volume criteria for certain surgical procedures and for care in a neonatal intensive care unit.

A fourth leap has since been added: a composite score from responses to a number of questions used to assess the hospital's culture of health.

From its founding in November 2000, the Leapfrog Group has grown to include 25 large corporate and trust purchasers and 34 business coalitions, and it has built formal liaisons with the Centers for Medicare & Medicaid Services, the Agency for Healthcare Research and Quality, and the Office of Personnel Management, which has oversight of health plans for all federal employees. A publicly available report features the scores of hospitals that have voluntarily reported their efforts on each of the leaps, and the website also displays the names of hospitals that are linked with Leapfrog but do not choose to report their results. Additionally, the Leapfrog Group publishes an annual report featuring comparative risk-adjusted resource utilization. Business coalitions have taken the key responsibility for implementing Leapfrog principles and local hospital reporting in their regions. The Leapfrog Group is important to members of hospital boards because the organization represents purchasers who wish to influence the marketplace using quality metrics that purchasers understand and that have direct relationships to reduced hospital mortality and morbidity rates.

## Impact of the Leapfrog Group

The Leapfrog Group has four major initiatives to help hospitals meet the growing demand for transparency in healthcare:

1. The Leapfrog Hospital Survey
2. Resource utilization report
3. The Leapfrog Group computerized provider order-entry comparative performance assessment
4. Leapfrog hospital rewards program

According to results from the 2009 Leapfrog Hospital Survey (2010), fewer than half of hospitals achieve adequate quality standards or acceptable standards for mortality. However, there has been some improvement: Of the 1,244 hospitals completing the 2009 survey, 53.5 percent met Leapfrog's quality standard for heart bypass surgery, compared to only 43 percent in 2008. Similarly, 44 percent of hospitals met Leapfrog's quality standard for heart angioplasty, compared to only 35 percent previously.

In 2009, less than 50 percent of hospitals met Leapfrog's outcome, volume, and process standards for six high-risk procedures and conditions (Exhibit 5.2). Research suggests that when hospital staff follow nationally endorsed and evidence-based guidelines for these procedures and conditions, lives are saved.

**Exhibit 5.2: Percentage of Reporting Hospitals That Fully Met Leapfrog's Standard in 2009**

**High-risk Surgery**

| | |
|---|---|
| Aortic valve replacement | 11.8% |
| Abdominal aortic aneurysm repair | 36.1% |
| Pancreatic resection | 33.5% |
| Esophageal resection | 31.5% |
| Weight-loss (bariatric) surgery | 36.6% |
| High-risk deliveries | 29.9% |

Waste also emerges as a problem. To gauge waste, Leapfrog's resource use measure is based on risk-adjusted mean length of stay tempered by readmission rates. Length of stay is a strong determinant of cost. In 2009, there was a 56 percent difference between the highest and lowest performing hospitals in resource use for heart bypass surgery. For heart angioplasty, there was a 79 percent difference between the highest and lowest performers.

Another innovation from the Leapfrog Group has been the testing of hospital computerized medication order-entry systems; computerized provider order entry (CPOE) simulation is part of the annual Leapfrog Hospital Survey. According to Leapfrog, 26 percent of the 1,244 hospitals that completed the survey in 2009 report having a CPOE system in at least one inpatient department. The Leapfrog Group unveiled a specific report on this topic in June 2010. Using a web-based simulation tool, 214 hospitals tested their CPOE systems for their ability to catch common medication errors, including errors that could lead to fatalities. The CPOE systems, on average, missed half of the routine medication orders and a third of the potentially fatal orders. Nearly all of the hospitals improved their performance after adjusting their systems and protocols and running the simulation a second time.

Leapfrog has also spurred development of an incentives program, currently in use by the state of Maine's employee benefits program. Hospitals are required to report data in order to participate. According to the Leapfrog CEO Leah Binder: "In states such as Maine, where participation and performance in the Leapfrog Hospital Survey are financially rewarded in the benefits package of one of the state's largest purchasers, we see larger margins of improvement year over year on both quality and resource use measures. Overall, where purchasers are actively using Leapfrog data, we see real change" (Leapfrog Group 2010).

The voluntary Leapfrog Hospital Survey results include 1,244 hospitals in 45 states. Individual hospital results can be viewed and compared at www.leapfroggroup.org/cp. The Leapfrog Group believes business interests and not the hospitals will propel the healthcare industry to embrace these changes at a faster pace.

## Future Issues for Hospital Boards

In the past decade, hospital board members have faced complex governance decisions in the marketplace. Declining revenues from Medicare and Medicaid have been paired with increasing numbers of uninsured. High-deductible health plan benefit designs have created large accounts receivable balances. Cost increases from multiple sectors in the industry and other cost drivers have created double-digit premium increases for private payers, including hospitals in their role as employers. Payers have responded by passing increasing healthcare costs to their employees. Concurrent with declining revenues, hospital board members are now confronted with new reporting and compliance requirements by purchasers and regulators. With the advent of the Patient Protection and Affordable Care Act, a new focus on reducing waste and adverse outcomes will further jeopardize the current revenue models. For example, payers such as Medicare and other businesses may not want to reimburse a hospital for avoidable errors or certain readmissions. Boards must now focus on margins per appropriate admission instead of number of beds filled and total bed days. Attaining high-quality, affordable service is indeed a daunting task.

Hospital board members can ask some basic questions about quality of care in their institution, such as the following:

- Do the board and administration have a collaborative working relationship with businesses and business coalitions in their community?
- Do board members know whether their institution's morbidity, mortality, and infection rates compare favorably with their peers locally and nationally?
- Is the institution more costly because of avoidable errors? For example, are pneumonia and heart attack patients staying longer because their first doses of necessary medication occur many hours after admission instead of within the first hour?
- Does hospital leadership provide this type of information to the board or to the community?

Future directions likely to be embraced by coalitions and their members will include the following:

- Support and encouragement of national standards and national organizations such as the National Quality Forum and the Leapfrog Group in addition to The Joint Commission
- Development of financial and nonfinancial incentives to improve/reward high-quality healthcare
- Required reporting to set benchmark performance requirements for hospitals in their communities and other sectors in healthcare
- Dissemination of this information to encourage wise purchasing and utilization decisions by businesses and by their employees
- Refusal to pay for waste, errors, and readmissions

Business coalitions are formed to lower healthcare costs to their members. In pursuit of this goal, they are dealing with local hospital leadership about both cost and quality. It is certainly the goal of both hospital boards and business coalitions to ensure the highest quality and most affordable hospital services for the benefit of all.

## Notes

1. Interested hospitals may contact IHI, which worked in 2003 on Hospital Standardized Mortality Rates (HSMR). IHI also has a white paper on mortality called "Move Your Dot." For more information, go to www.ihi.org.
2. Multiple websites publish hospital-specific information. One of the more widely trusted sites is hospitalcompare.hhs.gov, which uses Medicare data and features quality of care, mortality statistics, and patient satisfaction results. One commercial site that provides a variety of comparative hospital information is www.healthgrades.com.

## References

Berwick, D. "Request for Proposals: Replacing Don's Right Knee." 2003. Presented at the National Forum on Quality Improvement in Health Care, New Orleans, LA. December 3.

Codman, E. A. 1916. *A Study in Hospital Efficiency.* Boston: Th. Todd Co.

*Darling v. Charleston Community Memorial Hospital*, 33 Ill.2d 326, 211 N.E.2d 253, 14 A.L.R.3d 860 (Ill. Sep 29, 1965).

Dartmouth College. 2011. *Dartmouth Atlas of Healthcare.* www.dartmouthatlas.org

Eagle, K. A., C. K. Montoye, A. L. Riba, A. C. DeFranco, R. Parrish, S. Skorcz, P. L. Baker, J. Faul, S. M. Jani, B. Chen, C. Roychoudhury, M. A. C. Elma, K. R. Mitchell, and R. H. Mehta. 2005. "Guideline-Based Standardized Care Is Associated With Substantially Lower Mortality in Medicare Patients With Acute Myocardial Infarction." *Journal of the American College of Cardiology* 46 (7): 1242–48.

Institute for Healthcare Improvement. 2006. "5 Million Lives Campaign" Brochure.

Institute of Medicine Committee on Quality of Health Care in America. 2002. *Crossing the Quality Chasm: A New Health Care System for the 21st Century.* Washington, DC: National Academies Press.

Institute of Medicine Committee on Quality of Health Care in America. 2000. *To Err Is Human: Building a Safer Health System.* Washington, DC: National Academies Press.

The Leapfrog Group. 2010. "From the Leapfrog Hospital Survey: Quality Not Adequate and Waste a Major Problem." www.leapfroggroup.org/news/leapfrog_news/4775498.

———. 2003. "About Us." www.leapfroggroup.org/about_us.

McInnis, D. 2006. "What System?" *Dartmouth Medicine.* http://dartmed.dartmouth.edu/summer06/html/what_system.php.

Midwest Business Group on Health. 2003. "Reducing the Costs of Poor-Quality Health Care Through Responsible Purchasing Leadership." Chicago: Midwest Business Group on Health.

Mukherjee, D., J. Fang, S. Chetcuti, M. Moscucci, E. Kline-Rogers, and K. A. Eagle. 2003. "Impact of Combination Evidence-Based Medical Therapy on Mortality in Patients with Acute Coronary Syndromes." *Circulation* 109: 745–49.

National Business Coalition on Health. 2009. "NBCH Coalition Membership, State by State." www.nbch.org/index.asp?bid=67.

Reinertsen, J. 2011. "Questions to Ask When Forming a Board Quality Committee." Institute for Healthcare Improvement. www.ihi.org/knowledge/Pages/Tools/QuestionstoAskWhenForminagBoardQualityCommittee.aspx.

Vaughan, T., M. Koepke, E. Kroch, W. Lehrman, S. Sinha, and S. Levey. 2006. "Engagement of Leadership in Quality Improvement Initiatives: Executive Quality Improvement Survey Results." *Journal of Patient Safety* March (2): 2–9.

# CHAPTER SIX

# How to Provide Fiscal Oversight

*Dennis Stillman, University of Washington, Seattle*

## FINANCIAL OVERSIGHT

Ensuring the organization's financial health is the board's responsibility. To do this, management and the board must work together from their unique positions. The board approves financial objectives developed by management with the finance committee. Management prepares and provides understandable financial statements containing information the board finds useful. The finance committee and management look at detailed financial ratios, but all board members need to be conversant with the important components of the financial statements they receive.

## NECESSARY FINANCIAL INFORMATION

The board is responsible for ensuring the hospital's financial health in the near term and over time. The board does this by

1. approving financial objectives developed by management, including budgets, a long-range financial plan, and targeted credit rating.
2. seeing that strategic plans, capital investments, and budgets support the achievement of the approved financial objectives.
3. monitoring and assessing financial performance and requiring management to develop corrective actions when deficiencies are detected.
4. ensuring necessary internal controls are in place and functioning, overseeing the auditors, and ensuring financial statements are in accordance with generally

accepted accounting practices (GAAP) and accurately present the hospital's financial condition.

The first three of these responsibilities incorporate ratio analysis of the financial statements referred to in the fourth.

Financial statements are used by internal and external audiences to monitor and evaluate the financial condition of the hospital. The three primary financial statements are the *balance sheet, statement of operations,* and *statement of cash flow.*

## Balance Sheet

The balance sheet provides a snapshot of the hospital's financial condition on a specific date. On the left side or top of the balance sheet the reader finds assets (what is owned). Assets include cash, accounts receivable, buildings, and equipment. They are presented in decreasing order of liquidity. Assets that are or will be converted to cash within 12 months are categorized as current assets. Included in current assets are cash, accounts receivable, and inventory. Assets that will provide service over multiple years are categorized as noncurrent or long-term assets. These include buildings, equipment, and financial investments not intended to be consumed within 12 months.

On the right side or bottom of a balance sheet are the liabilities (what is owed to creditors) plus net assets or owner's equity (what the hospital is worth). Similar to assets, liabilities are sequenced in decreasing order of their expected settlement. Current liabilities will be paid within 12 months. These include payroll, accounts payable, and the current portion of long-term debt. The noncurrent or long-term liabilities are the amounts owed on loans with maturities greater than one year, including bonds payable and capital leases.

The net assets (for nonprofit organizations), or owner's equity (in for-profit hospitals), represent the accounting worth of the organization. If assets were sold for their listed values and all liabilities were paid, what remains would be the net assets available for distribution to the owners. Net assets are generated in several ways:

- Contributions by founders
- Transfers from a parent organization
- Sale of stock in commercial corporations
- Tax levy proceeds
- Retention of profits generated

The balance sheet reflects the basic accounting equation:

**Assets = Liabilities + Net assets**

The total assets must equal liabilities plus net assets. If you receive a balance sheet where total assets do not equal liabilities plus net assets, the accountants made an error.

## Statement of Operations

The second financial statement, the statement of operations, may be the most familiar. It presents information on how much revenue was earned and what expenses were incurred to generate the revenues. The excess of revenues over expenses is familiarly called *profit*. Profit is the fuel of the organization. It allows the hospital to develop new programs, enhance existing ones, and take risks. Other names for the statement of operations are profit and loss statement, revenue and expense summary, or income statement.

The statement of operations is prepared for a period of time ending on the date of the related balance sheet, such as "For the year ending December 31, 20X2" or "For the month ending December 31, 20X2." The statement includes all the revenues earned and expenses incurred during the covered period.

Net patient revenues are those earned from activities directly related to the hospital's primary business of patient care. They are valued at the estimated amounts to be collected, not at the prices charged. Premium revenues represent those generated when hospitals assume capitation risk versus being paid for services provided. Other operating revenues arise from activities indirectly related to patient care, such as cafeteria sales, parking fees, and research grants.

Nonoperating revenues are earned from sources not related to the core business of patient care. For most hospitals, investment income makes up the bulk of nonoperating revenues.

Operating expenses are the value of resources consumed to generate operating revenue. Major categories of expenses are

- Salaries and wages
- Benefits
- Supplies
- Purchased services
- Depreciation
- Provision for bad debts
- Interest expense

Operating revenues minus operating expenses equals net income from operations. This is what was earned from the primary business of patient care. Add nonoperating income to the net income from operations and you get net income, also called excess of revenues over expenses, the bottom line, or profit.

### Statement of Cash Flow

The statement of cash flow is the third common financial statement. It summarizes the cash inflows and outflows and links the cash balance on one balance sheet to the cash balance on the next one. Like the statement of operations, the statement of cash flows presents information for a period of time.

The statement of cash flows is broken out into three broad categories:

1. Cash flow from operating activities
2. Cash flow from investing activities
3. Cash flow from financing activities

Operating activities reflect the net cash flows in and out of the hospital from the regular operations of the hospital, patient services. Investing activities reflect cash flow from and to investments made in property, buildings, and equipment as well as financial investments, such as stocks and bonds. Financing activities show net cash flows from principal payments on long-term debt and proceeds from the sale of bonds and the issuance of stock. The financial statements combined provide an excellent basis for understanding the financial condition of a hospital.

## ANALYZING FINANCIAL STATEMENTS AND MONITORING FINANCIAL PERFORMANCE

Financial statements summarize the financial impact of thousands of events in the operation of a hospital. Using them to make judgments and assess the fiscal condition of an organization is difficult without further analysis. Exhibits 6.1, 6.2, and 6.3 are the balance sheet, statement of operations, and statement of cash flow for fictional Christopher Reid Hospital (CRH) covering 20X2 and 20X1. These statements will be used to illustrate financial ratio analysis.

# Exhibit 6.1: Balance Sheet

Christopher Reid Hospital
Balance Sheet
December 31, 20X2 and 20X1
(millions)

| ASSETS | 20X2 | 20X1 |
|---|---|---|
| **CURRENT ASSETS** | | |
| Cash | $ 114 | $ 77 |
| Marketable securities | 188 | 74 |
| Patient accounts receivable, net | 111 | 112 |
| Inventories | 14 | 13 |
| Other current assets | 21 | 19 |
| Total Current Assets | $ 448 | $ 295 |
| **LONG-TERM ASSETS** | | |
| Investments | 330 | 300 |
| Net property, plant & equipment * | $ 407 | $ 418 |
| Other long-term assets | 53 | 49 |
| Total Long-Term Assets | $ 790 | $ 767 |
| **TOTAL ASSETS** | $ 1,238 | $ 1,062 |

| LIABILITES & NET ASSETS | 20X2 | 20X1 |
|---|---|---|
| **CURRENT LIABILITIES** | | |
| Salaries, wages & related liabilities | $ 32 | $ 43 |
| Accounts payable & accrued expenses | 73 | 42 |
| Current portion of long-term debt | 9 | 8 |
| Total Current Liabilites | $ 114 | $ 93 |
| **LONG-TERM DEBT** | 349 | 295 |
| **TOTAL LIABILITIES** | $ 463 | $ 388 |
| **NET ASSETS** | | |
| Unrestricted | $ 767 | $ 666 |
| Restricted | 8 | 8 |
| Total Net Assets | $ 775 | $ 674 |
| **TOTAL LIABILITIES & NET ASSETS** | $ 1,238 | $ 1,062 |

| * | 20X2 | 20X1 |
|---|---|---|
| Property, plant & equipment | $ 856 | $ 820 |
| Less accumulated depreciation | $ 449 | $ 402 |
| Net property, plant & equipment | $ 407 | $ 418 |

**Exhibit 6.2: Statement of Operations**

Christopher Reid Hospital
Statement of Operations
Years Ended June 30, 20X2 and 20X1
(millions)

| | 20X2 | 20X1 |
|---|---|---|
| **Unrestricted Revenue** | | |
| Net patient service revenue | $ 815 | $ 793 |
| Premium revenue | 197 | 153 |
| Other operating revenue | 51 | 42 |
| **Total Unrestricted Revenue** | $ 1,063 | $ 988 |
| | | |
| **Expenses** | | |
| Salaries & wages | $ 366 | $ 354 |
| Employee benefits | 96 | 93 |
| **Total Labor Expenses** | $ 462 | $ 447 |
| Supplies | 161 | 166 |
| Purchased services | 158 | 141 |
| Depreciation | 53 | 51 |
| Provision for bad debts | 56 | 69 |
| Interest | 13 | 14 |
| Other | 74 | 67 |
| **Total Operating Expenses** | $ 977 | $ 955 |
| | | |
| **Operating Income** | $ 86 | $ 33 |
| **Nonoperating Income** | | |
| Investment income | 25 | 26 |
| | | |
| **Excess of Revenue over Expenses** | $ 111 | $ 59 |

The concept and calculation of a financial ratio is simple: One number is divided by another (and sometimes multiplied by 100 to produce a percentage).

$$\frac{\textbf{Numerator}}{\textbf{Denominator}} = \textbf{Ratio}$$

The numerator and denominator can be a single figure or a combination of them; they can be drawn from one financial statement or a combination of financial statements.

**Exhibit 6.3: Statement of Cash Flows**

Christopher Reid Hospital
Statement of Cash Flows
For the years ending December 31, 20X2 and 20X1

|                                          | 20X2       | 20X1      |
|------------------------------------------|-----------:|----------:|
| Cash flows from operating activities     | $    69    | $    40   |
| Cash flows from investing activities     | (86)       | (65)      |
| Cash flows from financing activities     | 54         | 30        |
| Net increase (decrease) in cash          | $    37    | $    5    |
| Cash balance, December 31, 20X1          | 77         | 72        |
| Cash balance, December 31, 20X2          | $   114    | $    77   |

Ratios are the indicators most frequently used by outsiders (such as bond rating agencies, lenders, and investors) to assess a hospital's financial condition and by insiders (boards and management) to monitor performance, plan, and make decisions. Ratio formulas are standardized, and benchmarks are available to assess an organization's financial condition and make comparisons with peer organizations.

There are four categories of financial ratios: liquidity, profitability, capital structure, and activity. Each takes its own look at an organization. Each section that follows will cover the following:

1. Introduce some commonly used ratios.
2. Show how they are calculated.
3. Illustrate them using CRH's 20X2 financial statements.
4. Briefly discuss what each means.
5. Compare CRH ratios to benchmark values. (The benchmarks used in this chapter represent typical values for a financially strong hospital in the late 2000s.)

## Liquidity Ratios

Liquidity ratios assess a hospital's ability to meet its short-term obligations (current liabilities) with its short-term resources (current assets). Most businesses that experience financial troubles do so because of liquidity problems—a lack of cash to pay debts as they come due.

### Current Ratio

The current ratio is the most basic measure of liquidity. It is calculated as

$$\frac{\textbf{Current assets}}{\textbf{Current liabilities}}$$

For CRH, that ratio is

$$\frac{\$448}{\$114} = 3.9$$

Both the numerator and denominator come from the balance sheet. This ratio measures how many times the current liabilities can be paid with (covered by) current assets. Current assets are considered "lazy" assets because they are not invested in producing services and thus do not generate revenues. Businesses want to hold as few of them as absolutely necessary, while maintaining the ability to meet short-term obligations as they come due.

CRH's current ratio is 3.9, indicating that for every dollar of current liabilities the hospital has $3.90 in current assets. The benchmark is 2.0; that is, current assets are twice the current liabilities. The prior year's current ratio value was 3.2. From a lender's standpoint, current ratios above the benchmark and upward trends are desirable; values below the benchmark and trends downward are undesirable. CRH's current ratio is above the benchmark, and the trend is increasing. Both are desirable.

### Days Cash on Hand

The days cash on hand is another liquidity ratio. It measures the number of days an organization could meet its average daily cash outlays with available cash and investments. It is typically calculated as:

$$\frac{\textbf{Cash + marketable securities + long-term investments}}{\textbf{(Operating expenses – depreciation – provision for bad debts)} \div \textbf{365}}$$

For CRH, the calculation is

$$\frac{\$114 + \$188 + \$330}{(\$977 - \$53 - \$56) \div 365 \text{ days}} = 266 \text{ days}$$

Cash, marketable securities, and long-term investments are found on the balance sheet; operating expenses, depreciation, and provision for bad debts are drawn from the statement of operations.

For 20X2, CRH's days cash on hand are 266 days; the benchmark is 198 and the prior year's was 197. The 20X2 days cash on hand are above the benchmark and the trend is increasing. Both are desirable.

Values above the benchmark and upward trends are desirable; values below the benchmark and decreasing trends are undesirable.

### Days in Accounts Receivable

Days in accounts receivable is a third liquidity ratio. It focuses on how long it takes to collect what it is owed (accounts receivable). This is a critical aspect of financial management. An organization's accounts receivable are constantly turning over. Services are provided to patients and accounts receivable increase. Bills are sent to payers and patients. Payments are received; accounts receivable are decreased, and cash is increased. Because accounts receivable are frequently a hospital's largest current assets, how they are managed should be closely monitored. This ratio is calculated as:

$$\frac{\textbf{Net patient accounts receivable}}{\textbf{(Net patient revenue} \div \textbf{365)}}$$

For CRH, the calculation is

$$\frac{\$111}{(\$815 \div 365 \text{ days})} = 50 \text{ days}$$

CRH's days in accounts receivable is 50 days; it takes about seven weeks from the time services are provided until the time the account is settled. The benchmark is 50 and the prior year's was 52 days. Thus, CRH collects about as rapidly as its peers, and it is getting better. Days in accounts receivable is closely tied to the amount of cash on hand. Here is an example: The average value of a day's worth of revenue is $2.2 million (net patient revenue ÷ 365). If CRH decreases its days in accounts receivable by 10 days with the receipt of cash, it would have an additional $22 million ($2.2 times 10 days) in its pocket rather than in the coffers of its payers. Additionally, if these funds could be invested at 4 percent interest, annual income would increase by more than $800,000.

Values of days in accounts receivable below the benchmark and declining trends are desirable; values above the benchmark and increasing trends are undesirable.

## PROFITABILITY RATIOS

Profits provide the means for a hospital to develop and grow. Absent an adequate level of profit, the organization must borrow more, its owners must invest more, donors must contribute more, or assets must be sold off. Profits are necessary for a hospital to have a future.

### EBITDA Margin

EBITDA (earnings before interest, taxes, depreciation, and amortization) margin measures profitability, including all sources of revenue (operating and nonoperating) and excluding interest expense, income taxes, and depreciations and amortization from expenses. It has become a commonly used ratio for hospitals in the last 10 years but has been used in other industries for much longer. It is calculated as

$$\frac{\text{Net income + Interest expense + Income taxes + Depreciation}}{\text{Total unrestricted revenue + Nonoperating income}}$$

For CRH, the calculation is
$$\frac{\$111 + \$13 + \$0 + \$53}{\$1,063 + \$25} \times 100 = 16.3\%$$

All of these values are taken from the statement of operations. Christopher Reid Hospital's EBITDA margin is 16.3 percent. The benchmark is 12.7 percent and the prior year's was 12.2 percent. CHR is performing better than its peers, and the trend is improving.

### Operating Margin

Operating margin is a more conservative measure of profitability. It includes only operating revenues and includes all operating expenses. It is calculated as:

$$\frac{\text{Net income from operations}}{\text{Total operating revenue}}$$

For CRH, the calculation is

$$\frac{\$86}{\$1,063} \times 100 = 8.1\%$$

All of these values are taken from the statement of operations. Christopher Reid Hospital's operating margin is 8.1 percent. The benchmark is 3.0 percent and the prior year's was 3.3 percent. CRH is performing better than its peers, and the trend is improving.

Hospitals have traditionally been thin-margin businesses. How much profit should a hospital earn? It needs to earn enough profit to implement its strategic plan or at least equal to the cost of capital.

Obviously, upward trends and values above the benchmark are desirable; the reverse is undesirable for both the EBITDA and operating margin ratios. CRH shows a strong trend and desirable variance from the benchmarks.

## Capital Structure Ratios

Capital structure focuses on the right side of the balance sheet and deals with the mix of lender- and owner-supplied funds, the amount of debt employed versus the amount invested by its owners (net assets or owners' equity).

### Debt to Capitalization

Debt to capitalization is a comparison of an organization's long-term debt to the sum of long-term debt and net assets. It is calculated as

$$\frac{\textbf{Long-term debt}}{\textbf{Long-term debt + Unrestricted net assets}}$$

For CRH, the calculation is

$$\frac{\$349}{\$1,116} \times 100 = 31.3\%$$

Both the numerator and denominator of this ratio are taken from the balance sheet. CRH's debt to capitalization ratio is 31.3 percent, meaning the hospital's creditors have lent about one-third of the capital used to fund the business. The ratio increases when an organization employs more borrowed funds, if net assets decrease because dividends are paid out (in for-profit hospitals), or if financial losses are experienced.

High values increase the difficulty and expense associated with securing additional long-term debt. The benchmark is 38 percent and the prior year's was 30.7 percent. CRH's value in 20X2 is below the benchmark and the trend is increasing slightly. It has a desirable comparison with the benchmark and an undesirable trend. These indicate that it still has capacity to take on some additional debt at relatively reasonable cost.

### EBITDA Coverage Ratio

EBITDA coverage ratio measures the ability of the organization to pay off (service) its debt. It is calculated as

$$\frac{\text{Net income + Interest expense + Income taxes + Depreciation}}{\text{Interest expense + Current portion of long-term debt}}$$

For CRH, the calculation is

$$\frac{\$111 + \$13 + \$0 + \$53}{\$13 + \$9} = 8.0 \text{ times}$$

Net income, interest expense, income taxes, and depreciation are taken from the statement of operations; principal payment on the long-term debt for the next year comes from the balance sheet—current portion of long-term debt.

CRH's EBITDA coverage ratio is 8.0 times, which means that it can pay the principal and interest on its long-term debt 8 times from its current performance; the benchmark is 4.4 times and the prior year's value was 5.6 times. CRH is comfortably above the benchmark, and the trend is also desirable. The key to maintaining this strength is strong profitability.

Values higher than the benchmark and increasing are desirable values; below the benchmark and declining are undesirable.

## Activity Ratios

Activity ratios focus on how well the hospital employs its assets to generate revenue (sales). Assets are resources; they can be deployed effectively or ineffectively to bring revenue into the business.

### Total Asset Turnover

Total asset turnover is a general measure of an organization's revenue-generating ability. It is calculated as

$$\frac{\text{Total operating revenues + Nonoperating revenues}}{\text{Total assets}}$$

For CRH, the calculation is

$$\frac{\$1,063 + \$25}{\$1,238} = 0.88 \text{ times}$$

Total operating revenue and nonoperating revenue are drawn from the statement of operations; total assets come from the left side of the balance sheet.

CRH ratio is 0.88 times, which indicates that 88 cents of revenue is generated for each dollar invested in assets. It is below the benchmark of 0.97 and below the previous year's value of 0.95. This implies that CRH is not using its assets as efficiently as its peers, nor its prior year.

Values above the benchmark and upward trends are desirable; lower values and downward trends are undesirable.

The denominator (total assets) can be deflated by old buildings and equipment (typically the largest component of assets), which increases the total asset turnover ratio. Conversely, newer assets (as well as more assets) can decrease the value.

This introduces us to our next ratio, average age of plant, to help us estimate the age of the hospital's buildings and equipment.

Average Age of Plant

Average age of plant is a way to estimate the accounting age of an organization's buildings and equipment. It is calculated as

$$\frac{\text{Accumulated depreciation}}{\text{Depreciation expense per year}}$$

For CRH, the calculation is

$$\frac{\$449}{\$53/\text{year}} = 8.5 \text{ years}$$

Accumulated depreciation comes from the balance sheet; depreciation expense is taken from the statement of operations. CRH's average age of plant is 8.5 years. The benchmark is 9.7 years and the prior year's value was 7.9 years, indicating that its assets are somewhat newer than those of its peers. This may indicate that it is technologically more current than its peers. Hospitals are capital-intensive businesses with rapid technological obsolescence. Remaining competitive requires state-of-the-art technology. This requires ongoing, carefully analyzed, and prioritized investments.

### Personnel Costs as a Percentage of Net Operating Revenues Ratio

Personnel are the most important resource hospitals apply in caring for patients. They also represent the largest category of costs of operating a hospital. The personnel cost as a percentage of net operating revenues quantifies this expenditure in relation to other resource utilization such as supplies. The ratio is calculated as

$$\frac{\textbf{Salaries and wages + Benefits}}{\textbf{Total operating revenue}} \times 100$$

For CRH, the calculation is

$$\frac{\$366 + \$96}{\$1,063} \times 100 = 43.5\%$$

Values below the benchmark and decreasing are desirable; values above the benchmark and increasing are undesirable.

CRH's ratio is 43.5 percent. The benchmark is 48.8 percent and the prior year's was 45.2 percent. It uses relatively fewer personnel than its peers and is continuing to make improvements on this performance.

## CONCLUSION

In summary, how is Christopher Reid Hospital doing financially based on our ratio analysis?

Overall, CRH is very strong financially with all but the total asset turnover ratio being better than the benchmark values (see Exhibit 6.4). The trends are also strong, except again for the total asset turnover and the average age of plant.

From the board's perspective, financial statement analysis provides a means of exercising financial oversight. Key aspects of the financial oversight role are:

1.  Select indicators of financial performance (for example, achieve ratio values consistent with an "A" bond rating).
2.  Specify ranges for these indicators within which they may vary.
3.  Measure actual performance against these indicators on a scheduled basis.

4. Depending on those results, celebrate accomplishments or expect action plans from management to correct the deficiencies.

The responsibilities of boards regarding financial performance are challenging. Financial statement analysis using financial ratios provides an excellent means to set objectives and monitor performance.

---

**Exhibit 6.4: Financial Ratio Table**

Christopher Reid Hospital
Financial Ratio Table

| | 20X2 | 20X1 | Benchmark | Compared to Benchmark | Trend |
|---|---|---|---|---|---|
| Current ratio | 3.9 | 3.2 | 2.0 | D | D |
| Days cash on hand | 266 | 197 | 198 | D | D |
| Days in accounts receivable | 50 | 52 | 50 | D | D |
| EBITDA margin | 16.3% | 12.2% | 12.7% | D | D |
| Operating margin | 8.1% | 3.3% | 3.0% | D | D |
| Debt to capitalization | 31.3% | 30.7% | 38.0% | D | D |
| EBITDA coverage | 8.0 | 5.6 | 4.4 | D | D |
| Total asset turnover | 0.88 | 0.95 | 0.97 | U | U |
| Average age of plant | 8.5 | 7.9 | 9.7 | D | U |
| Personnel cost as a percentage of operating revenues | 43.5% | 45.2% | 48.8% | D | D |

D = desirable
U = undesirable

---

# CHAPTER SEVEN

# How to Work with the Community

Today, expectations about ethical corporate responsibility have grown, in part due to the lack of corporate responsibility that has been demonstrated in several industries. Hospitals and healthcare systems are operating in this highly sensitive atmosphere and are being bombarded with messages that they owe more to society and must be more transparent and accountable. The community relations of a hospital or health system will be determined by the organization's relationship to its stakeholders and to the overall health status of the community in which it functions.

## STAKEHOLDERS
*Kenneth Bopp, clinical professor, Health Management & Informatics Group, University of Missouri, Columbia*

A hospital or healthcare system has a wide variety of stakeholders—individuals, groups, and other organizations that have a direct or indirect investment in the organization. They can affect or be affected by the hospital's actions, objectives, and policies. In light of the heightened sensibilities in corporate accountability, a hospital or healthcare system board must recognize that the links between the organization and its multiple stakeholders are increasingly critical to the organization's ability to maintain and enhance its reputation; its value and financial stability; and its ability to achieve its mission, vision, and goals. Knowledge about stakeholders is a critical source of competitive advantage.

## Stakeholder Identification

To begin, the hospital or healthcare system must first identify and understand who its stakeholders are. They include all the individuals and constituencies, both inside and outside the organization, who contribute either voluntarily or involuntarily to its value-creating capacity and activities and who are therefore its potential beneficiaries and/or risk bearers (Post, Preston, and Sachs 2002).

Stakeholders are also those individuals and organizations that are in a position to affect the organization's adoption of strategies and the implementation of decisions or actions. Thus, there is interdependency between the hospital or healthcare system and the stakeholders.

An organization's stakeholders can be categorized into three groups—internal, interface, and external stakeholders.

1. Internal stakeholders are people who operate entirely within the boundaries of the organization, including the management team, employees, and employed medical staff members.

2. Interface stakeholders function both internally and externally in relation to the organization, including the medical staff and joint-venture partners.

3. External stakeholders fall into three categories:

   • Those who provide inputs, including members or patients, third-party payers, volunteers, potential donors, and equipment and materials vendors
   • Those who compete with the organization for members, patients, and resources
   • Special interest groups concerned with how the organization's operations affect their specific interests. Examples of interest groups include investors (if applicable), economic development organizations, business and civic entities, the media, and governmental regulatory bodies

## Stakeholder Analysis and Management

In addition to the identification of the various stakeholders involved, the board should know the groups' values and concerns. An increasing regulatory climate and media attention to healthcare quality and safety have opened the door to a vast number of entities and people advocating for healthcare social responsibility issues.

Stakeholder analysis is the process of systematically gathering and analyzing qualitative information to determine which stakeholders need to be taken into account.

Stakeholder analysis will include the influence (i.e., the extent to which a stakeholder is able to affect the organization's outcomes) and the importance (i.e., the extent to which the stakeholder's problems, needs, and interest are affected by the organization's actions) of all identified stakeholders. Patterns will emerge to clarify which groups have the most relevance to the advancement of the hospital's mission, vision, and goals. Stakeholder analysis—the knowledge and understanding of an organization's stakeholders—is critical to stakeholder management.

## Stakeholder Importance, Concerns, and Exchange of Value with the Organization

The first requirement in developing an effective stakeholder strategy is for the governing board to recognize its role in managing this complex institutional responsibility. In the dispersed and multifaceted environment, hospitals and healthcare systems must collect information about reputational threats across the organization. The starting point is to put in place an effective early warning system to make the board and executive leadership aware of emerging reputational problems. Although hospitals and health systems' warning systems are good at tracking traditional media feeds, these systems must also monitor the multitude of web-based and social media, whose power is beginning to rival that of mainstream media.

When identifying stakeholders of influence, organizations should cast a broad net to include both traditional direct stakeholders (consumers, employees, shareholders, regulators) and indirect stakeholders (nongovernmental organizations and advocacy groups as well as the media), which help shape attitudes. Identified threats require an understanding of the issues that matter to the stakeholders and the degree to which the organization's activities affect the respective stakeholders' perceptions of the organization. This level of analysis requires a two-way dialogue to identify the perceptions of each kind of stakeholder and the root causes of their perceptions.

To begin, the stakeholder analysis worksheet in Exhibit 7.1 is a tool the board might use to assess the relative importance of its respective stakeholders, the stakeholder's concerns, and the mutual expectations and benefits of the respective relationships.

**Exhibit 7.1: Stakeholder Analysis Worksheet**

Stakeholder_____

1. Importance of stakeholder group:

   How large is the membership of this stakeholder group?_____
   How important is this stakeholder group to the organization?
   
   _____Very important
   _____Fairly important
   _____Neutral
   _____Not so important
   _____Not at all important

2. Concerns of the stakeholder group:

   What social, political, economic, health, or technical issue(s) is/are the primary concerns of the stakeholder?_____

3. Exchange of "value" between stakeholder group and the organization:

   a) Stakeholder expectations/perceptions of the organization?
   
   What does this group expect from the organization?
   
   _____
   
   How satisfied is this group with what it is getting from the organization?
   
   _____
   
   b) Organization's expectations/dependency on stakeholder group?
   
   What input does the organization receive from this group?
   
   _____
   
   To what extent is the organization dependent on this group?
   
   _____
   
   What does the organization expect from this group?
   
   _____
   
   How does this stakeholder group affect the organization's success or failure?
   
   _____

Organizations interested in a more in-depth assessment of the worth or threat of a potential or existing stakeholder relationship should ask the following additional questions:

1. What resources of the organization and each of its stakeholders are of value to the other?

2. What specific benefits will accrue to each stakeholder from its relationship with the other organization?
3. What specific benefits will accrue to the organization from its relationship with each stakeholder?
4. What risks will the organization face if it does not address the concerns of a specific stakeholder?
5. Do benefits outweigh the costs and risks of the relationship between the organization and the respective stakeholder?
6. What social value can be generated through the organization's relationship with the stakeholder?
7. What new resources, capabilities, and benefits can be created through the relationship with the respective stakeholder?
8. Has the organization's value creation and/or exchange with the respective stakeholder depreciated? If so, to what extent?
9. Can the organization's value construct with its respective stakeholder be renewed and enhanced for the benefit of both?

Responding to identified threats may require the board to increase transparency and actions to address the issues stakeholders value most. Reputations are built on a foundation not only of communication but also deeds. Stakeholders can see through public relations messages that are not supported by real and consistent organizational practices. Because a corporate reputation is based on stakeholder trust, demonstrated codes of conduct and integrity are essential to an organization's ability to share positive information with inside and outside stakeholders. Having demonstrated corporate social responsibility (CSR), organizations will be in a much better position to be transparent when there are legitimate deficiencies in CSR. Organizations can acknowledge they can do better and commit to taking corrective actions.

Although marketing and public relations play an important role in influencing stakeholders, these tools alone are insufficient in influencing stakeholders in today's interconnected world. Communication channels need to go beyond traditional PR approaches and emphasize two-way dialogue and face-to-face outreach to stakeholders, including social media, that can also play a crucial role in discussing CSR with stakeholders. As more and more consumers, bloggers, and organizations host interactive websites, brand image is moving out of the hands of organizations and traditional advertisers, giving stakeholders a different power in the marketplace. Consequently, two-way dialogue is critical. Underlying these priorities is a willingness to participate in the public debate more actively than many hospitals or health systems have in the past. Hospitals and health systems need to master this new forum and manage it, not just react to it.

Recent studies show rising consumer expectations for the role businesses play in society, but surveys find that only 6 percent of senior business leaders indicated their organizations were playing a leadership role in addressing social issues (Bonini 2010; Bonini, Court, and Marchi 2009). This gap between public expectations and the action of business leaders is also true of many healthcare organizations. The most widely known ways that CSR efforts create value is by enhancing the reputation of organizations through interactions with their stakeholders to increase their understanding of stakeholders' interest in, concerns about, and attitudes toward their organization's tangible CSR actions.

In the increasingly complex world of social responsibility and image, managing CSR successfully requires an integrated organizational approach many healthcare organizations lack. This makes it doubly important for the board and senior management to address CSR issues in their strategic planning. The involvement of the board and top leadership sends a strong signal to external stakeholders and the public, and their involvement is essential in creating the internal corporate culture. This motivates internal stakeholders to work across functional barriers to address these issues (Ayuso et al. 2007).

The healthcare board must shift its focus from a single organizational goal of wealth maximization to multiple objectives related to its diverse stakeholders (Meyer and Kirby 2010).

Board members both internal and external bring important links to stakeholders, but directors who currently have ties to the organization will be more motivated to focus internally (Hillman and Dalziel 2003). With regard to CSR, most recommendations favor the role of independent directors who may bring more external stakeholder relationships, knowledge, and legitimacy to the board and the organization's CSR efforts. Also, outside board members will be more likely than inside directors to oppose a narrow definition of organizational performance which focuses primarily on financial measures and will tend to be more sensitive to society's needs (Ibrahim and Angelidis 1995; Ibrahim, Howard, and Angelidis 2003). In addition, outside directors may be more knowledgeable about the changing demands of various stakeholders and feel freer to advocate costly and unpopular decisions, such as those that involve compliance issues (Johnson and Greening 1999). Kaufman and Englander (2005) recommend that a board that commits to CSR must have directors who can knowledgeably express the multiple constituents' interest in both ethical and economic terms. Thus, a board seeking to become more socially responsible may have to change its composition and functioning consistent with this new governance role. These governance recommendations call for more board independence and, in some instances, for increased board diversity and better response to stakeholders.

Each board will need to determine for itself how it will be involved as its community moves toward this new paradigm of stakeholder involvement. Each community will evolve at its own pace, and the hospital's board and management must not be caught napping as that occurs.

## HEALTH STATUS OF THE COMMUNITY
*Errol L. Biggs*

The debates over healthcare reform will continue to bring many proposals for improving quality of care and patient outcomes while curbing rising costs. And regardless of what happens with reform efforts, some prominent health system change leaders suggest existing healthcare organizations and their stakeholders must redesign their operations in a wide variety of ways (Lee 2010; Gawande 2010; Bohmer 2010; Levin-Scherz 2010). Admittedly, fixing healthcare and the health status of a community present formidable internal and external challenges for healthcare organizations and their boards.

For example, internal challenges may include healthcare professionals redesigning work processes across existing boundaries beyond the scope of the medical model and working as members of teams; shifting healthcare delivery from the current focus on episodic acute care to prevention and chronic condition management; and designing and implementing standardized care processes and protocols while knowing when and how to deviate from them. External challenges will likely involve reimbursement, laws and regulations, changing consumer expectations, and a variety of other sociological evolutions as discussed previously.

It appears that an organization's financial outcomes may depend, at least in part, on internal and external stakeholders' perception of the organization's reputation for environmental, social, and cultural programs that meet community needs and exceed regulatory requirements or industry norms. Moreover, in many other ways CSR programs can

- support growth (new markets, new customers, market share innovation),
- improve returns on capital (operational efficiency, workforce efficiency),
- reduce risk (mitigate problems with regulation, gain public support needed to do business, ensure the sustainability of supply chain), or
- improve management quality (leadership strength and development, adaptability of business, balance between short-term priorities and long-term strategic view) (Bonini, Koller, and Mirvis 2009).

On the other hand, healthcare institutions that are ignoring CSR issues should be made aware that this neglect may lead to consumer, public, or regulator backlash. Moreover, McKinsey surveys and experience suggest organizations that do not act on social and environmental issues could be forgoing other hard business benefits, such as access to new markets and workforce efficiency (Bonini, Koller, and Mirvis 2009). Some healthcare organizations have attempted to address public expectations through public relations initiatives or with token philanthropic or CSR programs. However, researchers have found that an organization cannot get credit for good deeds if it is struggling with ethics and governance issues, such as questions about how it treats customers or employees or concern about its behavior on social, economic, cultural or environmental issues where the public sees it as "part of the problem" (Bonini, Court, and Marchi 2009).

## Measuring Community Health Status

In the current atmosphere of corporate scrutiny, it is more important than ever for boards of hospitals and other healthcare organizations to actively monitor the health status of their communities. They should be aware of baseline information allowing them to determine if improvements are being made or if new problems are developing. Some organizations have even linked management compensation packages to measurable improvements in the health status of the community, sending a clear message that the board considers this area important.

An initial community health needs assessment and other surveys should be completed by management or a consulting firm to identify the baseline. On the hospital board, the quality and community health committee is usually responsible for reviewing the survey results and making recommendations to the board.

## Consumer Perception, Awareness, and Satisfaction Survey

Understanding how the community perceives the hospital or health system and its specific services or departments is important for strategic planning and positioning efforts. Respondents should be asked a series of questions about their satisfaction with past care and services provided by the organization and any area competitors. Compilation of quality and service satisfaction data helps providers assess how they are perceived by their constituents and by the community in general.

Many organizations are also interested in determining whether respondents would be interested in new services or products. Respondents should be asked to indicate how likely they or their family members would be to use a specific new service or program if it became available. This type of research can reduce costs and save staff time and energy by allowing focus on projects with the highest level of community interest. During this portion of the study, respondents are also often asked if they are aware the organization offers certain programs and services. Low awareness may indicate the organization should increase its marketing efforts to improve or increase utilization and knowledge of its ability to meet the community's healthcare needs.

## General Health Indicators/Health Profile Study

A comprehensive assessment of the community's morbidity and mortality data should be conducted. With this study, epidemiological data are analyzed and evaluated to determine major causes of death and illness in the community. Morbidity, mortality, and demographic data are compared to state and national data, and similarities and variances are identified and analyzed. Some communities have much lower or higher incidences of mortality and morbidity from certain diseases. Knowing what illnesses are affecting the health and longevity of the organization's community is critical to service planning and development. The types of data collected from secondary sources include demographic data, health status indicators, perinatal indicators, mortality data, morbidity data, and sociodemographic indicators.

## Population-wide Patterns of Health Services Use and Health Needs Assessment

Information about population-wide patterns of use and care needs is collected, usually through telephone surveys of randomly selected members in the target area. These surveys are designed to identify issues associated with access, affordability, and availability of healthcare services. They also obtain information about the healthcare needs of the population, patterns of healthcare service use, participation in risky lifestyles, and knowledge of managed care programs and insurance.

Healthcare organizations can then use this information to develop preventive health services and programs with the objective of improving the overall well-being of the community. This type of research methodology also involves reviewing health provider assessments, diagnosed and self-reported diseases, lifestyle risk factors, and demographic identifiers.

## Community Health Needs Assessment

Upon completion of the consumer perceptions and awareness surveys, the general health indicators study/health profile, and the population-wide health services use and health needs assessment, a comprehensive report should be submitted to management (if management did not conduct them) and to the quality and community health committee of the board. The report should provide an analysis of all study results and synthesize those results into a series of conclusions and recommendations. Based on the findings, management and/or the quality and community health committee will make recommendations to the board regarding new service or program development, community perceptions and attitudes about care, and community health needs activities. Key long- and short-term strategic planning issues will also be addressed.

The board's job is to review highlights and key indicators of improvement in the community's health status, as surveyed by management and the quality and community health committee, and to act on the recommendations.


## CONCLUSION

Healthcare organizations need broad legitimacy in the community where they operate if they are to sustain their long-term ability to create shareholder or nonprofit organizational value. Equally important, society depends on healthcare organizations to improve population health as well as to create environmental, social, economic, and cultural benefits to their communities. This relationship forms the basis of an overarching contract between hospitals and health systems and society. Responses to the social, environmental, and governance concerns of regulators, advocacy groups, consumers, and other stakeholders will continue to reshape the core businesses of the healthcare industry and individual healthcare entities.

As this reshaping continues, hospitals and health systems are increasingly challenged with transparency, the need to pull open the curtains revealing everything from quality, safety, and costs of service to the treatment of workers as well as how they address societal developments. There is also an increased need to determine the baseline from which the hospital will measure its progress and against which it will determine what community needs it should strategically plan to meet.

Increased social responsibility and community leadership means that healthcare organizations must be prepared to be viewed and held accountable in a manner different from how they have historically been viewed. Boards can be reactive and negative as they experience this new social accountability, or they can be proactive and take leadership and ownership of these new strategic opportunities. They may need to develop a mission and strategic position around CSR with appropriate performance metrics related to indirect and direct stakeholder issues. CSR calls for strategic and tactical actions on issues that matter most to stakeholders. Finally, CSR calls for an ongoing, often two-way, dialogue with stakeholders while balancing a CSR public image with maintaining the bottom line. Achieving CSR reputation may seem like using a lot of organizational resources and energy, but in today's climate, with reputational issues threatening the bottom line and the ability to achieve broader goals, a degree of high-level attention and integration is essential.

## References

Ayuso, S., M. A. Rodrigues, R. Garcia, and M. A. Arino. 2007. "Maximizing Stakeholders' Interests: An Empirical Analysis of the Stakeholder Approach to Corporate Governance." IESE Working Paper WP No 670.

Bohmer, R. M. J. 2010. "Fixing Health Care on the Front Lines," *Harvard Business Review* 88 (4): 62–69.

Bonini, S. 2010. "Toward Meeting Consumer Expectations." *McKinsey Quarterly* 1 (June) 100–101.

Bonini, S., D. Court, and A. Marchi. 2009. "Rebuilding Corporate Reputations." McKinsey Quarterly. www.mckinseyquarterly.com/Rebuilding_corporate_reputations_2367.

Bonini, S., T. M. Koller, and P. H. Mirvis. 2009. "Valuing Social Responsibility Programs." *McKinsey Quarterly* 4: 66.

Gawande, A. 2010. "Medicine Needs a New Kind of Hero." *Harvard Business Review* 88 (4): 60–61.

Hillman, A. J., and T. Dalziel. 2003. "Boards of Directors and Firm Performance: Agency and Resource Dependence Perspectives." *Academy of Management Review* 28 (3): 383–96.

Ibrahim, N. A., and J. P. Angelidis. 1995. "The Corporate Social Responsiveness Orientation of Board Members: Are There Differences Between Inside and Outside Directors?" *Journal of Business Ethics* 14 (5): 405–10.

Ibrahim, N. A., D. P. Howard, and J. P. Angelidis. 2003. "Board Members in the Service Industry: An Empirical Examination of the Relationship Between Corporate Social Responsiveness Orientation and Directional Type." *Journal of Business Ethics* 47 (4): 393–401.

Johnson, A. R., and D. W. Greening. 1999. "The Effects of Corporate Governance and Institutional Ownership Types of Corporate Social Performance."

*Academy of Management Journal* 42 (5): 564–76.

Kaufman, A., and E. Englander. 2005. "A Team Production Model of Corporate Governance." *Academy of Management Executive* 19 (3): 9–22.

Lee, T. H. 2010. "Turning Doctors into Leaders." *Harvard Business Review* 88 (4): 50–58.

Levin-Scherz, J. 2010a. "Five Reasons Why Costs Are So High and How to Tackle Them." *Harvard Business Review* 88 (4): 71–72

———. 2010b. "Premium Price, Poor Performance." *Harvard Business Review* 88 (4): 70.

Meyer, C., and J. Kirby. 2010. "Leadership in the Age of Transparency." *Harvard Business Review* 88 (4): 39–46.

Post, J. E., L. E. Preston, and S. Sachs. 2002. "Managing the Extended Enterprise: The New Stakeholder View." *California Management Review* 45 (1): 6–28.

# CHAPTER EIGHT

# The Board and Nonconventional Medicine

*Sita Ananth, director of Knowledge Services, Samueli Institute*

## COMPLEMENTARY AND ALTERNATIVE MEDICINE

Over the last decade, the number of Americans using nonconventional approaches to healthcare has been growing steadily. Known as complementary and alternative medicine (CAM), these modalities cover a spectrum of approaches ranging from ancient systems such as traditional Chinese medicine and ayurveda from India to more modern approaches, such as homeopathy.

The integration of CAM into existing programs and treatments in today's hospitals is growing. Board members need to be aware of this movement to determine if they wish their hospital to use CAM therapies and to what degree.

Complementary interventions are used *in conjunction with* conventional medicine. Alternative therapies are used *in place of* conventional medicine. An example of a *complementary therapy* is using acupuncture to treat nausea caused by chemotherapy. An example of *alternative medicine* may involve the use of a special diet to treat cancer instead of using surgery, radiation, or chemotherapy as recommended by a conventional physician. *Integrative healthcare* describes the combination of mainstream medical therapies and CAM therapies for which there is, in most cases, scientific evidence of safety and effectiveness.

According to data gathered by the National Institutes of Health's National Center for Complementary and Alternative Medicine (NCCAM), four out of ten Americans were seeking CAM in 2007 (Barnes, Bloom, and Nahin 2008). Following are some interesting facts and figures to think about (Eisenberg et al. 1998):

- People who chose CAM approaches were seeking ways to improve their health and well-being or to relieve symptoms associated with chronic, even terminal, illnesses or the side effects of conventional treatments.

- Commonly used CAM therapies included nonvitamin, nonmineral, natural products; deep breathing exercises; meditation; prayer; chiropractic care; yoga; massage; and diet-based therapies.
- CAM was most often used to treat back pain or back problems, head or chest colds, neck pain or neck problems, joint pain or stiffness, and anxiety or depression.
- CAM use was more prevalent among women, adults with more education, those who engaged in leisure-time physical activity, and among adults who had one or more existing health conditions or who made frequent medical visits in the prior year.
- The number of annual visits to CAM practitioners was 697 million—60 percent more than all primary care physician office visits combined. Patients spent $12–$19 billion on providers and a total of $34–$40 billion on CAM services and products combined.

### Forces Driving the Use of CAM

- Dissatisfaction with the current system and the belief that the interventions work and can make a difference (Berman and Straus 2004).
- People taking personal responsibility for their health, reevaluating therapeutic options, and adopting a practical lifestyle (Thorne et al. 2002).
- Greater public access to health information through resources available on the Internet and in journals, books, and organizations devoted to this field.
- The public's desire for personalized and patient-centered care rather than therapy-centered care.
- A proven effectiveness in dealing with many of the chronic diseases aging baby boomers are now facing.

### Meaning of CAM to Hospitals and Health Systems

A growing number of US consumers are demanding their hospitals offer more than traditional allopathic health services, wanting integrated CAM therapies into the care available in the hospital. In response, hospitals have been looking to satisfy the demands of their communities, but they are also looking at the vast amount of money currently being spent on CAM by their patients. Additionally, hospitals increasingly realize the vast majority of this potential revenue is out of pocket, self-pay from their clients/patients.

In a 2007 survey of approximately 6,000 hospitals in the United States regarding their delivery of CAM services, some fascinating data emerged (Ananth 2007):

- Almost 25 percent of hospitals offered one or more CAM modalities (up from 8 percent in 1998).
- CAM services were twice as likely to be provided in an outpatient setting than in an inpatient setting.
- Massage therapy, acupuncture, relaxation therapy, and meditation were the most popular outpatient services.
- Pet therapy, massage therapy, music and art therapy, and guided imagery were most commonly offered on an inpatient basis.
- Patient demand was the primary motivator for offering these services; other motivators were clinical effectiveness, attracting new patients, and differentiating a hospital from its competitors.
- More than half the responding hospitals stated that offering CAM services reflected their organizational mission.
- The majority of CAM services offered in hospitals were fee-for-service and were paid out of pocket by patients.
- The primary challenges facing hospitals in implementing successful CAM programs included physician resistance, lack of budget, lack of internal expertise, and provider credentialing.

Board members should be aware of the following issues:

- More than 70 percent of patients withhold information about their CAM use from their physicians (Eisenberg 1997). Physicians must be trained to ask for this information from patients so that they are knowledgeable about their patients' total health status. This is also an important patient safety and liability issue for hospitals, particularly with regard to negative drug–herb interactions.
- Clinicians need to be better educated about CAM. Providers' general concerns about using CAM therapy in practice stem from lack of knowledge about CAM therapy or a belief that CAM therapy is not effective or can do harm (Segal 2002).
- Lack of coordination is rampant. Physicians and CAM practitioners do not necessarily communicate with each other about their patients.

### What Board Members Need to Do

- Ascertain the community's interest in CAM. What would the public like to see offered in the hospital?
- Request a board education session about CAM so that all board members can learn more about the various modalities.
- Survey hospital employees to find out what hidden skills and interests they have related to CAM therapies.
- Learn more about what CAM services, if any, are being offered in your hospital. Are these efforts being supported by your CEO?
- Experience a few modalities, such as massage or acupressure, to understand how and why these work.

## GLOSSARY OF COMPLEMENTARY AND ALTERNATIVE MEDICINE TERMS

**Acupressure** is based on the principles of acupuncture. This ancient Chinese technique involves using finger pressure on specific points along the body to treat ailments.

**Acupuncture** is a treatment within traditional Chinese medicine (TCM), a system of healing that dates back thousands of years. At the core of TCM is the notion that the life force *qi* flows through energetic pathways (meridians) in the body. The proper flow of *qi* is thought to create health. An imbalance of *qi* (too much, too little, or a blocked flow) results in disease. Acupuncture needles are inserted at points along the meridians to restore the balance and flow of the *qi*.

**Alexander technique** is a method of therapeutic practices and body movements, such as proper posture and energy-efficient habits, that improve health, conserve energy, and reduce pain.

**Allopathic or conventional medicine** is medicine as practiced by holders of MD (medical doctor) or DO (doctor of osteopathy) degrees and by allied health professionals, such as physical therapists, psychologists, and registered nurses. Other terms for conventional medicine include allopathy, allopathic medicine, Western medicine, mainstream medicine, orthodox medicine, regular medicine, and biomedicine.

**Anthroposophic medicine** is a medical system that takes into account the spiritual and physical components of illness. A treatment regimen may include herbal and homeopathic medicines and dietary recommendations, art therapy, movement therapy, massage, and specially prepared baths.

**Aromatherapy** is the use of essential oils from plants for healing purposes. The oils are typically inhaled or absorbed through the skin as a treatment for infections and stress.

**Ayurveda** is the Sanskrit word for the science of life. Ayurveda is considered the oldest healing science and has been practiced in India for more than 5,000 years. The basic principle of ayurveda is the prevention of illness by maintaining balance in the body, mind, and spirit through proper diet and lifestyle habits. A chief aim of ayurveda, which is designed to help people live long and healthy lives, is to cleanse the body of substances that cause disease.

**Bioenergetics** holds that repressed emotions and desires affect the body and psyche by creating chronic muscular tension and diminished vitality and energy. Through physical exercises, breathing techniques, verbal psychotherapy, or other forms of emotional-release work, the therapist attempts to loosen the "character armor" and restore natural well-being.

**Biofeedback** is a technique that involves training the mind so that a person can improve his or her health by learning to control certain internal bodily processes that normally occur involuntarily, such as heart rate, blood pressure, muscle tension, and skin temperature. These activities can be measured with electrodes and displayed on a monitor, providing feedback to the participant about the internal workings of his or her body. The person is then taught techniques to gain control over "involuntary" activities.

**Breathwork** involves a variety of techniques that use patterned breathing to promote physical, mental, and spiritual well-being. Some techniques use the breath in a calm, peaceful way to induce relaxation or manage pain, whereas others use stronger breathing to stimulate emotions and emotional release.

**Chelation therapy** is a series of intravenous injections of the synthetic amino acid ethylenediaminetetraacetic acid to detoxify the body. The treatment often is used to treat arteriosclerosis, or hardening of the arteries.

**Chiropractic** is a form of diagnosing and treating illnesses that affect the nerves, muscles, bones, and joints of the body through spinal manipulation. One of the oldest healing practices, spinal manipulation was first described by Hippocrates in ancient Greece. More recently, Daniel David Palmer founded the current field of chiropractic in 1895, when he cured a man of deafness and acute back pain by realigning a displaced vertebra in his back. Although the practice of contemporary chiropractic now includes other interventions, spinal manipulation remains the essence of chiropractic.

**Cognitive behavioral therapy** is a well-studied psychotherapy that treats anxiety, depression, and other medical conditions, such as persistent pain, stress-related illness, chronic fatigue, and rheumatoid arthritis. Considered one of the principal mind–body modalities, it focuses on how positive thinking and action engender health.

**Complementary and alternative medicine (CAM)** is a group of diverse medical and healthcare systems, practices, and products that are not generally considered to be part of conventional medicine, such as acupuncture, massage therapy, herbal supplements, and others.

**Craniosacral therapy** is a manual therapeutic procedure used to remedy distortions in the structure and function of the craniosacral mechanism: the brain and spinal cord, the bones of the skull, the sacrum, and interconnected membranes. The procedure is used to treat chronic pain, migraine headaches, temporomandibular joint disease, and other conditions and is performed by a range of licensed health practitioners.

**Cure** is an externally applied medical intervention that removes all evidence of the diagnosed disease.

**Dance/movement therapies** use expressive movement as a therapeutic tool for personal expression and psychological or emotional healing. Practitioners work with individuals who have difficulties resulting from conditions such as physical disabilities, addictions, histories of sexual abuse, and eating disorders.

**Disease** is the diagnosis that derives from the patient's presenting signs, symptoms, and laboratory tests.

**Energy medicine** uses therapies involving "energy fields," such as healing touch and Reiki, that are based on the concept that human beings are infused with a subtle form of energy. This vital energy or life force is known under different names in different cultures, such as *qi* in traditional Chinese medicine (TCM), *mana* in Hawaiian medicine, *ki* in the Japanese Kampo system, and *prana* in ayurvedic medicine. Practitioners of energy medicine believe that illness results from disturbances of these subtle energies.

**Feldenkrais** is a therapy that combines movement training, gentle touch, and verbal dialogue to help create more efficient movement. In individual hands-on sessions, the practitioner's touch is used to address the student's breathing and body alignment along with a series of slow, nonaerobic motions.

**Feng shui** is the ancient Chinese practice of configuring home or work environments to promote health, happiness, and prosperity. Feng shui consultants may advise clients to make adjustments in their surroundings from color selection to furniture placement to promote a healthy flow of chi, or vital energy.

**Flower essences** are intended to alleviate negative emotional states that may contribute to illness or hinder personal growth. Drops of a solution infused with the captured essence of a flower are placed under the tongue or in a beverage. The practitioner helps the client choose appropriate essences, focusing on the client's emotional state rather than on a particular physical condition.

**Guided imagery** involves using mental images to promote physical healing or changes in attitudes or behavior. Practitioners may lead clients through specific visualization exercises or offer instruction in using imagery as a self-help tool. Guided imagery is often used to alleviate stress and to treat stress-related conditions such as insomnia and high blood pressure. The therapy also is used by persons with cancer, AIDS, chronic fatigue syndrome, and other disorders with the aim of boosting the immune system.

**Healing** is the process of recovery, repair, and return to wholeness. In this context, healing is a unique and personal process and experience that may or may not involve curing.

**Healing touch** is used by nurses and other practitioners to accelerate wound healing, relieve pain, promote relaxation, prevent illness, and ease the dying process. The practitioner uses gentle touch or works with his or her hands near the client's body in an effort to restore balance to the client's energy system.

**Herbal medicine** also called botanical medicine or phytomedicine, refers to the use of any plant's seeds, berries, roots, leaves, bark, or flowers for medicinal purposes. There is a rich heritage of herbal medicine in healing systems throughout the world. In addition, important drugs used in Western medicine, such as digitalis, the cancer chemotherapy drug vincristine, and ephedrine, have all been developed through research on medicinal herbs.

**Holistic medicine** is a healing philosophy that views a patient as a whole person, not as just a disease or a collection of symptoms. In the course of treatment, holistic medical practitioners may address a client's emotional and spiritual dimensions and the nutritional, environmental, and lifestyle factors that may contribute to an illness.

**Holistic nursing** is embraced by registered or licensed nurses who seek to care for the body, mind, and spirit of the patient. Some holistic nurses work in independent practices, offering primary and chronic care that incorporates a variety of alternative methods, from homeopathy to therapeutic touch.

**Homeopathy** is a medical system that uses minute doses of natural substances called remedies to stimulate a person's immune and defense systems. A remedy is chosen individually for a sick person based on its capacity to cause, if given in overdose, physical and psychological symptoms similar to those a patient is experiencing.

**Hypnotherapy** uses an altered, relaxed state of mind resembling sleep, but one in which a person can still concentrate, to help people change their awareness and intentions. Hypnotherapy is often used to help people learn to control bad habits, pain, and stress.

**Illness** is the human experience of a disease such as the manifestation of the patient's beliefs, fears, and expectations. Illness also includes the patient's influence on the cause, meaning and the course of the disease.

**Integrative medicine** is a multidisciplinary system of care that incorporates both biomedical and complementary therapies.

**Magnetic therapy** (also known as magnetic field therapy or biomagnetic therapy) involves using magnets, magnetic devices, or magnetic fields to treat a variety of physical and emotional conditions, including circulatory problems, certain forms of arthritis, chronic pain, sleep disorders, and stress. Treatments may be applied by a practitioner or as part of a self-care program.

**Massage therapy** has been practiced as a healing therapy for centuries in nearly every culture around the world. It helps relieve muscle tension, reduce stress, and evoke feelings of calmness by using touch to influence the activity of the musculo-skeletal, circulatory, lymphatic, and nervous systems.

**Mind–body medicine** is an approach to healing that uses the power of thoughts and emotions to positively influence physical health. As Hippocrates stated, "the natural healing force within each one of us is the greatest force in getting well."

**Meditation** refers to a myriad of practices that relax the body and calm the mind. In particular, mindfulness-based stress reduction (MBSR), an approach based on a Buddhist meditation practice, is now used widely to relieve stress and enhance well-being.

**Naturopathic medicine** emphasizes the curative power of nature and treats acute and chronic illnesses in all age groups. Naturopathic physicians work to restore and support the body's own healing ability using a variety of modalities including nutrition, herbal medicine, homeopathic medicine, and Asian medicine.

**Nutrition** is the study of the relationship between food and physical health. More specifically, it is the science of nutrients and how they are digested, absorbed, transported, metabolized, stored, and discharged by the body. Clinical nutrition also includes the study of how the environment affects the quality and safety of foods and how these factors influence health and disease.

**Osteopathy** is a complete system of medical care. Its underlying philosophy is to treat the whole person, not just the person's symptoms. Osteopathy emphasizes the interrelationships of structure and function and the appreciation of the body's ability to heal itself. Osteopathic manipulation is one of the major components of this medical system.

**Qigong** is a traditional Chinese medicine practice that uses movement, affirmations, breath work, visualizations, and meditation to improve the flow of *qi* or life force and to restore both external and internal harmony.

**Reiki** is an ancient Tibetan healing system that uses hand placements to channel healing energies to the recipient. Although practitioners may vary widely in technique and philosophy, Reiki commonly is used to treat emotional and mental distress and chronic and acute physical problems, and to assist the recipient in achieving spiritual focus and clarity.

**Relaxation techniques** are helpful tools for coping with stress and promoting long-term health by regulating the body's autonomic nervous system and quieting the mind. Techniques that are used to induce relaxation, or used in conjunction with relaxation techniques, include meditation, guided imagery, yoga, breathing exercises, hypnosis, and others. Used daily, these practices can, over time, lead to a healthier response to stress.

**Spiritual healing** is practiced by healers who often regard themselves as conductors of healing energy or sources from the spiritual realm. They may call on spiritual helpers, such as power animals, angels, inner teachers, the client's higher self, or other spiritual forces. These forms of healing can be used as part of treatment for a range of emotional and physical illnesses.

**Spirituality** is defined as belief in a power operating in the universe that is greater than oneself, a sense of interconnectedness with all living creatures, and an awareness of the purpose and meaning of life. Medical systems such as traditional Chinese medicine, ayurveda, and Native American medicine include the development of increased spirituality as part of their health-promoting strategies. Recently, the power of prayer and other spiritual practices have been explored in medical settings.

**Tai chi** is a gentle exercise program derived from the martial arts. A traditional Chinese medicine practice, tai chi is composed of slow, deliberate movements, meditation, and deep breathing, which enhance physical health and emotional well-being.

**Therapeutic touch** is practiced by registered nurses and others to relieve pain and stress. The practitioner assesses where the person's energy field is weak or congested and then uses his or her hands to direct energy into the field to balance it.

**Traditional Chinese medicine (TCM)** is a complete medical system that has been used to diagnose, treat, and prevent illnesses for more than 2,000 years. TCM is based on a belief in yin and yang or opposing energies, such as male and female, winter and summer, and happiness and sadness. When yin and yang are in balance, a person is energized. Out of balance, however, yin and yang negatively affect health and well-being. In TCM, this state of balance is achieved through multiple approaches including herbal medicines, acupuncture, and qigong.

**Trigger point myotherapy** is a therapy in which pressure is applied by a practitioner to specific points on the body to relieve tension. Trigger points are tender, congested spots on muscle tissue that may radiate pain to other areas. Though the technique is similar to shiatsu or acupressure, this therapy uses Western anatomy and physiology as its basis.

**Yoga** is a spiritual practice that uses physical postures, breathing exercises, and meditation to improve overall health and well-being. Yoga began nearly 6,000 years ago in India as part of the classical healing science known as ayurveda.

**Yoga therapy** uses yoga to address mental and physical problems while integrating body and mind. Practitioners work one-on-one or in group settings, assisting clients with yoga postures, sometimes combined with therapeutic verbal dialogue.

**Zero balancing** is a method for aligning body structure and body energy. Through touch akin to acupressure, the practitioner seeks to overcome imbalances in the structure/energetic interface of the body, which is said to exist beneath the level of conscious awareness. Zero balancing is often used for stress reduction.

## References

Ananth, S. 2007. "Complementary and Alternative Medicine Survey of Hospitals." www.healthforum.com.

Barnes, P. M., B. Bloom, and R. L. Nahin. 2008. "Complementary and Alternative Medicine Use Among Adults and Children: United States, 2007." National Health Statistics Reports; no 12. Hyattsville, MD: National Center for Health Statistics.

Berman, J. D., and S. E. Straus. 2004. "Implementing a Research Agenda for Complementary and Alternative Medicine." *Annual Review of Medicine* 55: 239–54.

Eisenberg, D. 1997. "Advising Patients Who Seek Alternative Medical Therapies." *Annals of Internal Medicine* 127: 61–69.

Eisenberg, D. M., R. B. Davis, S. L. Ettner, S. Appel, S. Wilkey, M. Van Rompay, and R. C. Kessler. 1998. "Trends in Alternative Medicine Use in the United States, 1990-1997: Results of a Follow-up National Survey." *Journal of the American Medical Association* 280 (18): 1569–75.

Segal, L. 2002. "Views and Use of Complementary and Alternative Medicine by Mid-Atlantic Permanente Medical Group Health Care Providers." *Permanente Journal* 6 (4).

Thorne, S., B. Paterson, C. Russell, and A. Schultz. 2002. "Complementary/Alternative Medicine in Chronic Illness as Informed Self-Care Decision Making." *International Journal of Nursing Studies* 39 (7): 671–83.

# Epilogue

As trustees of all hospitals and healthcare systems know, being a board member today is much more difficult than it was even five years ago, and it could become even more difficult in the future. With healthcare reform, expansion of parts of Sarbanes-Oxley to include nonprofits, much higher interest in measuring quality and clinical outcomes, and changing reimbursements, boards are facing challenging times.

The increasingly turbulent overall business environment has caused an increased focus on boards of directors in general, including those in healthcare. Just as boards in the public sector are receiving amplified scrutiny, communities and key stakeholders are watching to see if nonprofit boards are building long-term value and structuring themselves to make appropriate decisions while providing needed services to the community in a cost-effective, clinically sound, and efficient manner.

In this environment, healthcare boards must consciously review their structure and assess how they work. This book has been designed to help a hospital or health system board function effectively to achieve its organizational vision. It can be used as a guide by new board members and for review by continuing members. It can be used in part or as a whole. Some components will fit certain hospitals more than others; most of the information, however, has universal application.

Directors who structure their boards for the long term will be more effective than their counterparts that do not. To function smoothly for the benefit of their hospitals, boards should have:

- Appropriate job descriptions
- A defined member-selection process
- A good orientation program
- Continuing education programs

- An effective committee structure
- A process to monitor quality
- A defined stakeholder analysis process
- An effective board–CEO relationship
- A thorough self-assessment process
- An understanding of everyone's roles and responsibilities
- A continuing desire to relate to their key stakeholders and communities.

The ideal governing board of a healthcare organization will be one that has looked at the information and recommendations in this book, decided which will improve its performance, and made the changes that fit. The effective healthcare board should strive to reach consensus and harmony with its employees, its community, and its key stakeholders. If just one strategy in this book helps accomplish that, it is worthwhile. Good luck!

—Errol L. Biggs

# Sample Conflict of Interest Policy

*Gregory Piche, Singularity Legal, Denver, Colorado, and the Office of the Attorney General, State of Minnesota.*

[name of hospital or health system]
## CONFLICT OF INTEREST POLICY

## SECTION 1. PURPOSE:

_____ is a nonprofit, tax-exempt organization. Maintenance of its tax-exempt status is important both for its continued financial stability and for public support. Therefore, the IRS as well as state regulatory and tax officials view the operations of _____ as a public trust, which is subject to scrutiny by and accountable to such governmental authorities as well as to members of the public.

Consequently, there exists between _____ and its board, officers, and management employees and the public a fiduciary duty, which carries with it a broad and unbending duty of loyalty and fidelity. The board, officers, and management employees have the responsibility of administering the affairs of _____ honestly and prudently, and of exercising their best care, skill, and judgment for the sole benefit of_____. Those persons shall exercise the utmost good faith in all transactions involved in their duties, and they shall not use their positions with _____ or knowledge gained therefrom for their personal benefit. The interests of the organization must be the first priority in all decisions and actions.

## SECTION 2. PERSONS CONCERNED:

This statement is directed not only to directors and officers, but to all employees who can influence the actions of _____. For example, this would include all who make purchasing decisions, all persons who might be described as "management personnel," and anyone who has proprietary information concerning _____.

## SECTION 3. AREAS IN WHICH CONFLICT MAY ARISE:

Conflicts of interest may arise in the relations of directors, officers, and management employees with any of the following third parties:

1. Persons and firms supplying goods and services to _____.
2. Persons and firms from whom _____ leases property and equipment.
3. Persons and firms with whom _____ is dealing or planning to deal in connection with the gift, purchase or sale of real estate, securities, or other property.
4. Competing or affinity organizations.
5. Donors and others supporting _____.
6. Agencies, organizations. and associations which affect the operations of _____.
7. Family members, friends, and other employees.
8. Proprietary or political interests associated with all or a _____ segment of the medical staff.

## SECTION 4. NATURE OF CONFLICTING INTEREST:

A conflicting interest may be defined as an interest, direct or indirect, with any persons or firms mentioned in Section 3. Such an interest might arise through:

1. Owning stock or holding debt or other proprietary interests in any third party dealing with _____.

2. Holding office, serving on the board, participating in management, or being otherwise employed (or formerly employed) with any third party dealing with _____.

3. Receiving remuneration for services with respect to individual transactions involving _____.

4. Using _____'s time, personnel, equipment, supplies, or good will for other than _____-approved activities, programs, and purposes.

5. Receiving personal gifts or loans from third parties dealing or competing with _____. Receipt of any gift is _____ is disapproved except gifts of a value less than $50, which could not be refused without discourtesy. No personal gift of money should ever be accepted.

6. Owning stock or holding debt or other proprietary interest in any _____ third party in direct competition with any service line of _____.

## SECTION 5. INTERPRETATION OF THIS STATEMENT OF POLICY:

The areas of conflicting interest listed in Section 3, and the relations in those areas which may give rise to conflict, as listed in Section 4, are not exhaustive. Conflicts might arise in other areas or through other relations. It is assumed that the directors, officers, and management employees will recognize such areas and relation by analogy.

The fact that one of the interests described in Section 4 exists does not necessarily mean that a conflict exists, or that the conflict, if it exists, is material enough to be of practical importance, or if material, that upon full disclosure of all relevant facts and circumstances it is necessarily adverse to the interests of _____.

However, it is the policy of the board that the existence of any of the interests described in Section 4 shall be disclosed before any transaction is consummated. It shall be the continuing responsibility of the board, officers, and management employees to scrutinize their transactions and outside business interests and relationships for potential conflicts and to immediately make such disclosures.

## SECTION 6. DISCLOSURE POLICY AND PROCEDURE:

Transactions with parties with whom a conflicting interest exists may be undertaken only if all of the following are observed:

1. The conflicting interest is fully disclosed.
2. The person with the conflict of interest is excluded from the discussion and approval of such transaction.
3. A competitive bid or comparable valuation exists; and
4. The [board or a duly constituted committee thereof] has determined that the transaction is in the best interest of the organization.

Disclosure in the organization should be made to the chief executive officer (or if she or he is the one with the conflict, then to the board chair), who shall bring the matter to the attention of the [board or a duly constituted committee thereof]. Disclosure involving directors should be made to the board chair (or if she or he is the one with the conflict, then to the board vice-chair), who shall bring these matters to the [board or a duly constituted committee thereof].

The [board or a duly constituted committee thereof] shall determine whether a conflict exists and in the case of an existing conflict, whether the contemplated transaction may be authorized as just, fair, and reasonable to _____ . The decision of the [board or a duly constituted committee thereof] on these matters will rest in their sole discretion, and their concern must be the welfare of _____ and the advancement of its purpose.

# Sample Conflict of Interest Disclosure Statement

*Gregory Piche, Singularity Legal, Denver, Colorado, and the Office of the Attorney General, State of Minnesota.*

## CONFLICT OF INTEREST DISCLOSURE STATEMENT

Preliminary note: In order to be more comprehensive, this statement of disclosure/questionnaire also requires you to provide information with respect to certain parties that are related to you. These persons are termed "affiliated persons" and include the following:

a. Your spouse, domestic partner, child, mother, father, brother or sister;

b. Any corporation or organization of which you are a board member, an officer, a partner, participate in management or are employed by, or are, directly or indirectly, a debt holder or a beneficial owner of any class of equity securities; and

c. Any trust or other estate in which you have a substantial beneficial interest or as to which you serve as a trustee or in a similar capacity.

1. **Name of employee or board member: (Please print)**

   _____

2. **Capacity:**

   _____ board of directors
   _____ executive committee         _____ committee member
   _____ officer                     _____ staff (position):

   _____

3. Have you or any of your affiliated persons provided services or property to _____ in the past year?

_____Yes _____No

If yes, please describe the nature of the services or property and, if an affiliated person is involved, the identity of the affiliated person and your relationship with that person:

_____

_____

_____

4. Have you or any of your affiliated persons purchased services or property from _____ in the past year?

_____Yes _____No

If yes, please describe the purchased services or property and, if an affiliated person is involved, the identity of the affiliated person and your relationship with that person:

_____

_____

_____

5. Please indicate whether you or any of your affiliated persons had any direct or indirect interest in any business transaction(s) in the past year to which _____ was or is a party?

_____Yes _____No

If yes, describe the transaction(s) and if an affiliated person is involved, the identity of the affiliated person and your relationship with that person:

_____

_____

_____

6. Were you or any of your affiliated persons indebted to pay money to _____ at any time in the past year (other than travel advances or the like)?

_____Yes _____No

If yes, describe the transaction(s) and if an affiliated person is involved, the identity of the affiliated person and your relationship with that person:

_____

_____

_____

7. In the past year, did you or any of your affiliated persons receive, or become entitled to receive, directly or indirectly, any personal benefits from _____ or as a result of your relationship with _____, that in the aggregate could be valued in excess of $1,000, that were not or will not be compensation directly related to your duties to _____?

_____Yes          _____No

If yes, please describe the benefit(s) and, if an affiliated person is involved, the identity of the affiliated person and your relationship with that person:

_____

_____

_____

8. Are you or any of your affiliated persons a party to or have an interest in any pending legal proceedings involving _____?

_____Yes          _____No

If yes, please describe the proceeding(s) and, if an affiliated person is involved, the identity of the affiliated person and your relationship with that person:

_____

_____

_____

9. Please indicate whether you or any of your affiliated persons have any direct or indirect competition financial interest in any company or venture  in direct competition with any service line of _____.

_____Yes          _____No

If yes, please identify the company or venture and describe the interest to which you refer.

_____

_____

_____

10. Please indicate whether you have any personal, professional or social relationship with any person or group associated with or affiliated with _____ that would prevent you from acting at all times in the best interests of _____.

_____Yes                    _____No

If yes, please identify the relationship and concern.

_____

_____

_____

11. Are you aware of any other events, transactions, arrangements or other situations that have occurred or may occur in the future that you believe should be examined by _____'s [board or a duly constituted committee thereof] in accordance with the terms and intent of _____'s conflict of interest policy?

_____Yes                    _____No

If yes, please describe the situation(s) and, if an affiliated person is involved, the identity of the affiliated person and your relationship with that person:

_____

_____

_____

I HEREBY CONFIRM that I have read and understand _____'s conflict of interest policy and that my responses to the above questions are complete and correct to the best of my information and belief. I agree that if I become aware of any information that might indicate that this disclosure is inaccurate or that I have not complied with this policy, I will notify [designated officer or director] immediately.

_____          _____
Signature                                  Date

# Sample Board Member
# Performance Appraisal, Short Version

[name of hospital or health system]
## BOARD MEMBER ANNUAL PERFORMANCE APPRAISAL

Completed by the Governance Committee and Communicated by
Board Chair or Governance Committee Chair
(Short Version)

| Assessment | Exceeds Expectation | Meets Expectation | Below Expectation |
|---|---|---|---|
| **A. Director is current in knowledge and understanding of the following:** | | | |
| 1. Mission and goals | _____ | _____ | _____ |
| 2. Hospital's priorities | _____ | _____ | _____ |
| 3. Hospital's financial status | _____ | _____ | _____ |
| 4. Quality of care issues. | _____ | _____ | _____ |
| **B. Director has been able to devote sufficient time to board responsibilities, including reviewing and analyzing board materials before each meeting.** | | | |
| | _____ | _____ | _____ |
| **C. Director regularly attends board meetings and actively participates.** | | | |
| | _____ | _____ | _____ |

*(continued)*

| Assessment | Exceeds Expectation | Meets Expectation | Below Expectation |
|---|---|---|---|

**D. Director's skill set is relevant to current competitive environment.**

| | _____ | _____ | _____ |

**E. Director has satisfactory working relationships with the board chair, other board members, and CEO.**

| | _____ | _____ | _____ |

_____          _____
Director                                             Date


_____          _____
Chair                                                Date
(Board or Governance
Committee)

# Sample Board Member
# Performance Appraisal, Long Version

(Name of Organization)

## BOARD MEMBER ANNUAL PERFORMANCE APPRAISAL

Completed by Governance Committee and Communicated by Board Chair
or Governance Committee Chair
(Long Version)

|  | Limited (1) | Acceptable (2) | Expected (3) | Impressive (4) | Exemplary (5) |
|---|---|---|---|---|---|
| **1. Commitment:** | | | | | |
| a. Prepares for meetings | ____ | ____ | ____ | ____ | ____ |
| b. Regularly attends board meetings | ____ | ____ | ____ | ____ | ____ |
| c. Reads materials and participates in board education programs | ____ | ____ | ____ | ____ | ____ |
| **2. Understands role:** | | | | | |
| a. Knows appropriate organizational channels of operation | ____ | ____ | ____ | ____ | ____ |
| b. Considers other viewpoints | ____ | ____ | ____ | ____ | ____ |
| c. Willing to compromise | ____ | ____ | ____ | ____ | ____ |

*(continued)*

| | Limited (1) | Acceptable (2) | Expected (3) | Impressive (4) | Exemplary (5) |
|---|---|---|---|---|---|
| **3. Decision making:** | | | | | |
| a. Strives for necessary information | _____ | _____ | _____ | _____ | _____ |
| b. Willing to make decisions with less than total information when necessary | _____ | _____ | _____ | _____ | _____ |
| c. Takes appropriate risks | _____ | _____ | _____ | _____ | _____ |
| d. Supports board decisions | _____ | _____ | _____ | _____ | _____ |
| e. Challenges decisions, with cause | _____ | _____ | _____ | _____ | _____ |
| **4. Analytical skills:** | | | | | |
| a. States issues and problems clearly and concisely | _____ | _____ | _____ | _____ | _____ |
| b. Conclusions reflect good judgment and thoughtful evaluation | _____ | _____ | _____ | _____ | _____ |
| c. Understands results of decisions | _____ | _____ | _____ | _____ | _____ |
| d. Opinions and comments reflect adequate knowledge of healthcare industry | _____ | _____ | _____ | _____ | _____ |
| **5. Dependability:** | | | | | |
| a. Follows through on commitments | _____ | _____ | _____ | _____ | _____ |
| b. Reports and projects are on time | _____ | _____ | _____ | _____ | _____ |
| **6. Personal traits:** | | | | | |
| a. Remains poised under stress | _____ | _____ | _____ | _____ | _____ |
| b. Tactful | _____ | _____ | _____ | _____ | _____ |
| c. Appropriate appearance | _____ | _____ | _____ | _____ | _____ |
| d. Gets along with people | _____ | _____ | _____ | _____ | _____ |
| e. Sensitive to others' feelings | _____ | _____ | _____ | _____ | _____ |
| **TOTAL** | _____ | _____ | _____ | _____ | _____ |

## GRAND TOTAL

_____  22–44  Limited

_____  45–66  Acceptable

_____  67–88  Expected

_____  89–110  Impressive

_____  111–120  Exemplary

**Action taken:** _____

_____

_____

_____

_____

_____

# Sample CEO Employment Contract

American College of Healthcare Executives. 2010. *Employment Contracts for Healthcare Executives: Rationale, Trends, and Samples,* 5th ed. Chicago: Health Administration Press.

## MODEL CHIEF EXECUTIVE OFFICER EMPLOYMENT CONTRACT (LONG FORM)

This agreement, made and effective as of the ___ day of _____, 20XX, between [name of Healthcare Organization], a corporation and [name of CEO].

WHEREAS, the Healthcare Organization desires to secure the services of the CEO and the CEO desires to accept such employment.

NOW THEREFORE, in consideration of the mutual covenants contained in this Agreement, and intending to be legally bound, the Healthcare Organization and the CEO agree as follows:

1. The CEO will render full-time services to the Healthcare Organization in the capacity of Chief Executive Officer of the corporation. The CEO will at all times, faithfully, industriously and to the best the CEO's ability, perform all duties that may be required of him by virtue of his position as Chief Executive Officer and all duties set forth in Healthcare Organization bylaws and in policy statements of the Board. It is understood that these duties shall be substantially the same as those of a chief executive officer of a business corporation. The CEO shall have and shall perform any special duties assigned or delegated to him by the Board.

2. In consideration for these services as Chief Executive Officer, the Healthcare Organization agrees to pay the CEO a base salary of $_____ per annum or such higher figure as shall be agreed upon at an annual review of his compensation and performance by the Board. This annual review shall occur three months prior to the end of each year of the contract for the express purpose of considering increments. Salary shall be payable in accordance with the payroll policies of the Healthcare Organization. The CEO may elect to defer such portion of his salary to the extent permitted by law in accordance with policies established by the Healthcare Organization.

3. (a)   The CEO shall be entitled to _____ days of paid time off for vacation and sick leave each year, to be taken at times agreed upon by the Chairman of the Board.

   (b)   In the event of a single period of prolonged inability to work due to the results of a sickness or an injury, the CEO will be compensated at his full rate of pay for at least _____ months from the date of the sickness or injury.

   (c)   In addition, the CEO will be permitted to be absent from the Healthcare Organization during working days to attend business and educational meetings and to attend to such outside duties in the healthcare field as have been agreed upon by the Chairman of the Board. Attendance at such approved meetings and accomplishment of approved professional duties shall be fully compensated service time and shall not be considered vacation time. The Healthcare Organization shall reimburse the CEO for all expenses incurred by the CEO incident to attendance at approved professional meetings, and such entertainment expenses incurred by the CEO in furtherance of the Healthcare Organization's interests; provided, however, that such reimbursement is approved by the Chairman of the Board.

   (d)   In addition, the CEO shall be entitled to all other fringe benefits to which all other employees of the Healthcare Organization are entitled.

4. The Healthcare Organization agrees to pay dues to professional associations and societies and to such service organizations and clubs of which the CEO is a member, approved by the Chairman of the Board as being in the best interests of the Healthcare Organization.

5. The Healthcare Organization also agrees to:

(a) insure the CEO under its general liability insurance policy for all acts done by him in good faith as Chief Executive Officer throughout the term of this contract;

(b) provide, throughout the term of this contract, a group life insurance policy for the CEO in an amount equivalent to $_____, payable to the beneficiary of his choice;

(c) provide comprehensive health and major medical insurance for the CEO and his family;

(d) purchase travel accident insurance covering the CEO in the sum of $_____;

(e) furnish, for the use of the CEO, an automobile, leased or purchased at the beginning of alternate fiscal years, and reimburse him for expenses of its operation; and

(f) contribute on behalf of the CEO to a retirement plan qualified under the Internal Revenue Code, at the rate of $____ per month.

6. The Board may, in its discretion, terminate this Agreement and the CEO's duties hereunder. Such action shall require a majority vote of the entire Board and become effective upon written notice to the CEO or at such later time as may be specified in said notice. After such termination, the Healthcare Organization shall continue to pay the CEO's then monthly base salary for the month in which his duties were terminated and for 24 consecutive months thereafter as an agreed upon severance payment. During this period, the CEO shall not be required to perform any duties for the Healthcare Organization or come to the Healthcare Organization. Neither shall the fact that the CEO seeks, accepts, and undertakes other employment during this period affect such payments. Also, for the period during which such payments are being made, the Healthcare Organization agrees to keep the CEO's group life, health, and major medical insurance coverage paid up and in effect and the CEO shall be entitled to outplacement services offered by the Healthcare Organization. The severance arrangements described in this paragraph will not be payable in the event that the CEO's employment is terminated due to the fact that the CEO has been charged with any felony criminal offense, or any misdemeanor criminal offense related to substance abuse, healthcare fraud or abuse, violent crimes, sexual misconduct, crimes involving children or the operation of the Healthcare Organization, or has been excluded from Medicare, Medicaid, or any other Federal Healthcare Program.

7. Should the Board in its discretion change the CEO's duties or authority so it can reasonably be found that the CEO is no longer performing as the Chief

Executive Officer of the Healthcare Organization and/or its parent corporation, the CEO shall have the right, within 90 days of such event, in his complete discretion, to terminate this contract by written notice delivered to the Chairman of the Board. Upon such termination, the CEO shall be entitled to the severance payment described in Paragraph 6, in accordance with the same terms of that Paragraph.

8. If the Healthcare Organization is merged, sold, or closed, the CEO may, at the CEO's discretion, terminate this Agreement or be retained as President of the Healthcare Organization, or any successor corporation to or holding company of the Healthcare Organization. If the CEO elects to terminate his employment at such time, he shall be entitled to the same severance arrangement as would be applicable under Paragraph 6 if the Healthcare Organization had terminated his employment at such time. Any election to terminate employment under this Paragraph must be made prior to the Healthcare Organization's merger, sale or closure, as applicable. If the CEO elects to continue to be employed by the Healthcare Organization or its successor organization, all of the terms and conditions of this Agreement shall remain in effect. The Healthcare Organization agrees that neither it nor its present or any future holding company shall enter into any agreement that would negate or contradict the provisions of this Agreement.

9. Should the CEO in his discretion elect to terminate this contract for any other reason than as stated in Paragraph 7 or 8, he shall give the Board 90 days written notice of his decision to terminate. At the end of the 90 days, all rights, duties and obligations of both parties to the contract shall cease and the CEO will not be entitled to severance benefits.

10. If an event described in Paragraphs 6, 7, or 8 occurs and the CEO accepts any of the severance benefits or payments described therein, the CEO shall to the extent not prohibited by law be deemed to voluntarily release and forever discharge the Healthcare Organization and its officers, directors, employees, agents, and related corporations and their successors and assigns, both individually and collectively and in their official capacities (hereinafter referred to collectively as "Releasees"), from any and all liability arising out of employment and/or the cessation of said employment. Nothing contained in this paragraph shall prevent the CEO from bringing an action to enforce the terms of this Agreement.

11. The CEO shall maintain confidentiality with respect to information that he receives in the course of his employment and not disclose any such information. The CEO shall not, either during the term of employment or thereafter, use or permit the use of any information of, or relating to the Healthcare

Organization in connection with any activity or business and shall not divulge such information to any person, firm, or corporation whatsoever, except as may be necessary in the performance of his duties hereunder or as may be required by law or legal process.

12. During the term of this employment and during the 24-month period following termination of his employment, the CEO shall not directly own, manage, operate, join, control, or participate in or be connected with, as an officer, employee, partner, stockholder, or otherwise, any other hospital, medical clinic, integrated delivery system, health maintenance organization, or related business, partnership, firm, or corporation (all of which hereinafter are referred to as "entity") that is at the time engaged principally or significantly in a business that is, directly or indirectly, at the time in competition with the business of the Healthcare Organization within the service area of the Healthcare Organization. The service area is defined as [DESCRIBE BY COUNTIES, ZIP CODES, A MILEAGE RADIUS, ETC.]. Nothing herein shall prohibit the CEO from acquiring or holding any issue of stock or securities of any entity that has any securities listed on a national securities exchange or quoted in a daily listing of over-the-counter market securities, provided that at any one time the CEO and members of the CEO's immediate family do not own more than 1 percent of any voting securities of any such entity. This covenant shall be construed as an agreement independent of any other provision of this Agreement, and the existence of any claim or cause of action, whether predicated on this Agreement or otherwise, shall not constitute a defense to the enforcement by the Healthcare Organization of this covenant. In the event of actual or threatened breach by the CEO of this provision, the Healthcare Organization shall be entitled to an injunction restraining the CEO from violation or further violation of the terms thereof.

13. The CEO shall not directly or indirectly through his own efforts, or otherwise, during the term of this Agreement, and for a period of 24 months thereafter, employ, solicit to employ, or otherwise contract with, or in any way retain the services of any employee or former employee of the Healthcare Organization, if such individual has provided professional or support services to the Healthcare Organization at any time during this Agreement without the express written consent of the Healthcare Organization. The CEO will not interfere with the relationship of the Healthcare Organization and any of its employees and the CEO will not attempt to divert from the Healthcare Organization any business in which the Healthcare Organization has been actively engaged during his employment.

14. Terms of a new contract shall be completed, or the decision made not to negotiate a new contract made, not later than the end of the tenth month. This contract and all its terms and conditions shall continue in effect until terminated.

15. This contract constitutes the entire agreement between the parties and contains all the agreements between them with respect to the subject matter hereof. It also supersedes any and all other agreements or contracts, either oral or written, between the parties with respect to the subject matter hereof.

16. Except as otherwise specifically provided, the terms and conditions of this contract may be amended at any time by mutual agreement of the parties, provided that before any amendment shall be valid or effective it shall have been reduced to writing and signed by the Chairman of the Board and the CEO.

17. The invalidity or unenforceability of any particular provision of this contract shall not affect its other provisions, and this contract shall be construed in all respects as if such invalid or unenforceable provision had been omitted.

18. This agreement shall be binding upon the Healthcare Organization, its successors and assigns, including, without limitation, any corporation into which the Healthcare Organization may be merged or by which it may be acquired, and shall inure to the benefit of the CEO, his administrators, executors, legatees, heirs and assigns.

19. This agreement shall be construed and enforced under and in accordance with the laws of the State of _____.

20. Any controversy, dispute or disagreement arising out of or relating to this Agreement, or the breach thereof, shall be settled by arbitration, which shall be conducted in _____, _____ in accordance with the American Health Lawyers Association Alternative Dispute Resolution Service Rules of Procedure for Arbitration, and judgment on the award rendered by the arbitrator may be entered in any court having jurisdiction thereof.

This contract signed this _____ day of _____, 200X.

[NAME OF HEALTHCARE ORGANIZATION]

WITNESS: _____ BY:_____
                                                          (Board Chair)
WITNESS: _____ _____
                                                          (Name of CEO)

# ACKNOWLEDGEMENT

## ANNOTATIONS TO CHIEF EXECUTIVE OFFICER CONTRACT

This contract is the "long form" CEO contract. It is somewhat more formal than the letter of agreement and specifically lays out some of the minimal benefits that a CEO should receive. Its formality and extensiveness make it more applicable as part of the negotiations for a new relationship than as a contract proposed during an existing one. It should be examined so that the items covered are raised in the negotiations rather than for the exact benefit and salary structure stated. Some benefits will be agreed upon and some not. That is the purpose of a contract negotiation.

## PARAGRAPH 1

This paragraph sets forth the duties of the Chief Executive Officer in very general terms. The specific duties of the CEO are not spelled out in the contract itself for two reasons. First, since the CEO should be involved in virtually every area of hospital operations, he must not be hamstrung by a limited "laundry list" of duties that narrowly circumscribe the scope of his responsibility. Such lists relegate the CEO to the status of a "hired hand." In addition, since the duties of the CEO constantly change as the organization changes, it is unwise to lock him and the Healthcare Organization into a set routine from the start. The contract likens the CEO's role to that of a CEO in a business corporation to underscore the broad responsibility entrusted with him.

## PARAGRAPH 2

This paragraph contains the financial terms of the contract, specifically, the CEO's salary. An annual figure is inserted in the first blank, while his monthly pay rate should be included in the second blank. The latter, of course, can be a weekly or bimonthly rate, depending on how the hospital or executive payroll is so structured. After each annual salary review, the CEO's salary will presumably increase. New salary levels should be contained in a letter to the CEO from the Board Chairman, which will become incorporated into the initial contract. By the contract language the CEO is also permitted the discretion to direct that a portion of his salary go into tax shelters as deferred income to the extent permitted by law.

## PARAGRAPH 3

This paragraph deals in general with compensation for time spent by the CEO away from the hospital, including vacation, sick leave and out-of-hospital business. An alternative to laying these benefits out in the contract is to include them in a separate letter agreement.

Subparagraph 3(a) deals with vacation time for the CEO. Vacation time is compensated at the CEO's full rate, and can be accumulated over the life of the contract.

Subparagraph 3(b) deals with sick leave in a similar fashion except that, unlike vacation time, it cannot be accumulated.

Subparagraph 3(c) deals with disability payments in the event of a major sickness or injury to the CEO. It can take the place of or supplement any disability insurance policy that the CEO may have in effect.

Subparagraph 3(d) permits the CEO to attend professional or hospital association meetings. The meetings to be attended should be agreed to in advance, or expense accounts approved after the fact by the Chairman of the Board. According to this clause, the CEO is entitled to reimbursement for all his expenses and for his full salary while in attendance at these meetings. Also, the travel expenses of the CEO's spouse and any necessary business entertainment expenses are also paid for. It should be stressed that the Chairman of the Board should approve all expense accounts of the CEO, for the CEO's own protection.

## PARAGRAPH 4

The CEO's dues for professional associations, service organizations or clubs that he belongs to are paid for by the Healthcare Organization, so long as his membership in them is reasonably related to the interests of the Healthcare Organization. It should not be necessary that these be approved in advance, but the Chairman of the Board should approve what organizations are joined by the CEO.

## PARAGRAPH 5

Subparagraph 5(a) requires the Healthcare Organization to include for coverage the CEO under its general liability insurance policy for any acts done by him in good faith during the course of his duties. This is absolutely essential since CEOs are very often named in lawsuits by patients alleging negligence or by physicians alleging that a denial or termination of medical staff appointment was improper. The Healthcare Organization must protect the CEO if he is to carry out his duties innovatively, aggressively and effectively.

The fringe benefit described in subparagraph 5(b) provides the CEO with a group life insurance policy, paid for by the Healthcare Organization. Of course, the CEO may name the beneficiaries of this policy. Subparagraphs 5(c) and (d), respectively, provide for comprehensive health insurance and travel accident insurance paid for by the Healthcare Organization. The health insurance package may be with Blue Cross/Blue Shield, a commercial carrier, or the Healthcare Organization's own self-insurance mechanism.

Subparagraph 5(e) provides for an automobile to be used by the CEO, the expenses of which are to be borne by the Healthcare Organization. Finally, subparagraph 5(f) permits payments into a retirement plan which are over and above the CEO's base of salary.

## PARAGRAPH 6

This clause is commonly referred to as the termination provision. It is by far the most important part of the Contract. In the event that a majority of the Board decides the services of the CEO are no longer required, for whatever reason, the contract is terminated. However, the CEO will still be entitled to a stated amount of salary even though he or she is no longer working for the Healthcare Organization. Also, the CEO's group life and health insurance benefits continue. Outplacement services are also made available. The exact number of months of severance pay to which the CEO is entitled is of course the subject of negotiation. The figure determined upon should accurately reflect the risks and challenges of the position.

However, this provision relieves the Healthcare Organization from its obligation to pay the severance arrangements in the event that the CEO's employment is terminated due to the CEO being charged with a criminal offense.

The purpose of this clause is to protect the CEO from threats of termination aimed at making him act in his position with unnecessary caution. It is in the interest of the Board, the Healthcare Organization and the patients. The CEO must be able to exercise his authority to the fullest extent possible. He must also be able to make hard decisions without fear that his job may be in jeopardy simply because someone on the Board or the medical staff did not like the choices he has made.

## PARAGRAPH 7

This paragraph is similar to Paragraph 6, except that it comes into play in the event that the Board substantially changes the duties of the CEO, either by appointing another officer with similar duties or by restricting the authority of the existing

CEO. This would be one way to avoid the applicability of the severance provisions of Paragraph 6. As in the case of Paragraph 6, the CEO will be entitled to full salary plus group life and health insurance benefits for two years after termination.

## PARAGRAPH 8

This paragraph provides for severance payments in the event of merger or closure of the Healthcare Organization.

## PARAGRAPH 9

This clause allows the CEO to voluntarily terminate the employment relationship, but if he does, no severance payment is made.

## PARAGRAPH 10

This paragraph protects the Healthcare Organization from needless future litigation by the CEO if the CEO accepts the severance benefits. This allows the Healthcare Organization to conduct its business relationship with the CEO without unnecessary caution. It is in the interest of the Board, the Healthcare Organization and the patients. This waiver will be enforced to the maximum extent allowable by law.

## PARAGRAPH 11

This provision protects the Healthcare Organization from disclosure of confidential information by the CEO during and after his term of employment with the Healthcare Organization. An employment contract with a key executive should contain a provision that prohibits the employee from disclosing to outsiders confidential information acquired by the employee during his term of employment without the express written permission of the employer. This provision should describe the applicable information so as to put the employee on notice as to what constitutes confidential information.

## PARAGRAPH 12

An employment contract with an executive employee typically contains a covenant by the employee not to compete with the employer during the term of the contract and for a specified period of time following termination of employment. The covenant is essential to the employer in order to prevent the employee from dealing with the employer's customers or otherwise engaging in competitive activities with the employer immediately following his termination of employment so as to cause material adverse financial consequences to the business of the employer.

Restrictive employment covenants have generally been held to be valid where the restraint imposed on the employee is no greater than necessary to protect the legitimate business interests of the employer, and where neither the hardship to the employee nor the likely injury to the public outweighs the employer's need for protection. Thus, a covenant not to compete is usually upheld if it is clearly and reasonably limited as to time and area, and does not extend beyond the duration and geographical scope necessary for the protection of the employer. It should be noted that such restrictive covenants are unenforceable in some states.

## PARAGRAPH 13

This provision prevents the CEO, whose employment at the Healthcare Organization has been terminated, for whatever reason, from recruiting other key executives to leave the Healthcare Organization and join him in independent ventures excluding the Healthcare Organization's involvement.

## PARAGRAPH 14

This paragraph makes it simple for the Healthcare Organization and the CEO to continue the agreement beyond its initial term by signing a simple letter of agreement as an extension. The letter need only state that the initial contract has been extended for another specified period and set out the CEO's new salary. All of the initial provisions and benefits continue in force during the extension.

## PARAGRAPH 15

This is a standard clause that appears in most contracts. It states that this particular contract embodies total agreement of the parties and supersedes any previous contract, in response to the so-called "parole evidence rule" of contract law. It eliminates any questions there may be as to the subject matter contained in the contract.

## PARAGRAPH 16

This provision requires that any amendments to the contract have to be stated in writing. This prevents either side from claiming that an "oral understanding" superseded some portion of this contract. It is technically referred to as a "no oral modification" or NOM clause.

## PARAGRAPH 17

This is known technically as a "savings clause." In the event that any portion of the contract is declared invalid or unenforceable by a court, the rest of the contract still remains in effect. The contract can therefore not be terminated on a "technicality."

## PARAGRAPH 18

This paragraph keeps the contract in force even though the hospital may change its corporate structure or be sold to another owner. It also provides that any benefits provided under the contract, such as life or accident insurance, that survive the CEO upon his death, inure to the benefit of his estate or heirs.

## PARAGRAPH 19

This clause stipulates what law applies to the contract. This is especially useful in hospitals near state lines. The law governing the contract should always be that of the state in which the hospital is located.

The execution of the contract should be authorized by the Board. It should be signed by the Chairman of the Board and the CEO, and should be witnessed by two individuals who are not on the Board and who are not members of the CEO's family. It should be filed along with other essential corporate documents. A copy should be given to the CEO. Needless to say, the terms of the contract, especially those relating to salary levels, fringe benefits and termination, should be treated as confidential.

# CEO Separation Agreement

American College of Healthcare Executives. 2010. *Employment Contracts for Healthcare Executives: Rationale, Trends, and Samples,* 5th ed. Chicago: Health Administration Press.

## SEPARATION AGREEMENT

### BY AND BETWEEN

[Name of Healthcare Organization], a nonprofit corporation organized under the laws of the State of _____ (hereinafter called the "Employer"),

### AND

[Name of Executive], an individual (hereinafter called "Executive").

### WITNESSETH:

WHEREAS, the Employer and Executive are parties to an Employment Agreement (the "Agreement") which was entered into on _____, 20___, the terms of which were partially modified by an Executive Severance Benefit Plan (the "Severance Plan") effective _____, 20___; and

WHEREAS, the Employer and Executive wish to set forth the terms of Executive's separation from employment and terminate the Agreement and the Severance Plan as specified herein.

NOW, THEREFORE, in consideration of the mutual covenants herein contained and intending to be legally bound hereby, the parties hereto agree as follows:

1. **Termination of Employment.**

   Executive shall cease to be employed by the Employer as of the close of business on _____, 20___ (the "Termination Date"). Except as expressly provided herein, the Employment Agreement, the Severance Plan, and all amendments thereto are expressly superseded by this Agreement upon its execution by both parties, and all rights and obligations of both parties pursuant thereto shall cease as of the Termination Date. As of _____, 20___, Executive shall no longer serve as President and Chief Executive Officer of the Employer or of any of its subsidiaries, shall no longer perform any duties, and shall not be authorized to act on behalf of the Employer or of any of its subsidiaries. Executive shall also cease to be an officer and a member of the Board of the Employer and of any other entities controlled by the Employer (collectively "Affiliates") as of the Termination Date.

2. **Payments and Benefits Upon Termination of Employment.**

   (a) Executive shall receive his Base Salary for a period of _____ (_____) months from the Termination Date, in accordance with the Employer's regular payroll practices and procedures, in effect from time to time, for senior management executives. "Base Salary" shall mean the total annual base salary payable to Executive at the rate in effect as of the Termination Date, which was _____ dollars ($_____) per annum. During this _____ (_____) month period, Executive shall not be required to perform any duties for the Employer or any Affiliate. Neither shall the fact that Executive seeks, accepts, and undertakes other employment during this period affect such payments. *In addition, the Employer has arranged for a senior executive outplacement program to assist Executive in securing another position, pursuant to the agreement with _____, which is attached as Exhibit _____.*

   (b) Executive's benefits listed on Exhibit A shall continue during the period when Executive receives severance pay hereunder to the extent that such continuation is permissible under controlling law (e.g., nondiscrimination or risk of forfeiture limitations) and benefit plan and policy provisions (as reasonably determined by the Employer). If a benefit cannot be continued, the Employer shall be released of its obligation to provide such benefit to Executive, and the Employer shall not be obligated to pay Executive any cash or other benefit in lieu of such noncontinued benefit. If the Employer changes the level of coverage or level of benefits under the plans for active employees during the benefit continuation period, the benefits for Executive shall be similarly modified. Executive shall also be entitled to extend said benefits at his own expense beyond the benefit continuation period as specifically provided for by the federal COBRA statute. Except as listed on Exhibit A, all other benefits shall be discontinued. Executive shall receive such distributions or conversion rights as may be provided for by applicable benefit plans.

(c) Executive shall also receive via direct payroll deposit on _____, 20___ $_____ as compensation for _____ hours of unused paid time off to which Executive is entitled under the employee benefit policies of the Employer.

(d) In accordance with the Employment Agreement, Executive shall be entitled to his share of any performance bonus pursuant to the Annual Incentive Plan for the President and Chief Executive Officer for FYE 20___ prorated to reflect the portion of the fiscal year that Executive was employed (i.e., _____/365, or _____% of Executive's full year share, if any).

(e) Payments to Executive under Sections 2(a), (b), (c), and (d) shall be subject to such withholdings for federal income taxes social security, Medicare, FUTA, state and local income, and other applicable taxes as may be required by law from time to time or higher amounts as may be designated by Executive in accordance with applicable laws or regulations.

3. **Company Property.**

Executive represents to the Employer that he has turned over to the Employer all cell phones, computers, PDAs, pagers, files, memoranda, records, other documents, keys, keycards, and any other physical or personal property of which he has possession, custody or control, which are the property of the Employer, *including the automobile that was leased by the Employer for the Employee's use.*

4. **Miscellaneous.**

(a) Subject to the non-competition clause contained in Section 6, Executive may seek employment elsewhere as of the Termination Date.

(b) The Employer will refer letters and phone calls that are personal to Executive to his home phone number and address as noted in his personnel file or to such other forwarding address as Executive may designate in writing.

## 5. Confidential Information.

Executive acknowledges that, by reason of his employment by the Employer, Executive has had access to confidential information and trade secrets of the Employer and its Affiliates, including, without limitation, information and knowledge pertaining to patients and patient lists, marketing strategies, business plans, managed care or other payor relationships (including but not limited to rate information), medical staff, pending or actual litigation, peer review matters, corporate compliance matters, personnel matters, vendor relationships, and all other confidential or proprietary information (collectively, "Confidential Information"). Executive agrees to maintain confidentiality with respect to Confidential Information that he received in the course of his employment and shall not disclose any such Confidential Information without the express written permission of the Board of the Employer. Executive shall not use or permit the use of any Confidential Information of or relating to the Employer or any Affiliates in connection with any activity or business and shall not divulge such Confidential Information to any person, firm, or corporation whatsoever, except as may be necessary in the performance of his duties hereunder or as may be required by law or legal process. The obligation of confidentiality imposed by this Section shall not apply to information that becomes generally known to the public through no act of Executive in breach of this Agreement. Further, in the event of any dispute concerning this Agreement, Executive may disclose to his attorney such Confidential Information as may be directly relevant to such dispute, or to the court subject to the terms of a confidentiality agreement, and protective order, reached by the parties and approved by the court.

## 6. Non-Competition.

(a) For a period of _____ (_____) months following the Termination Date, Executive shall not, unless acting pursuant hereto or with the prior written consent of the Board of the Employer, directly or indirectly own, manage, operate, finance, join, control, or participate in or be connected with, as an officer, director, employee, partner, principal, agent, representative, consultant, or otherwise, or use or permit Executive's name to be used in connection with: (i) any other hospital or health care facility, health system, or related business that is at the time engaged principally or significantly in a business that is, directly or indirectly, at the time in competition with the business of the Employer or any Affiliate and within the service area of the Employer or any Affiliate, or (ii) any entity doing business with the Employer or any Affiliate within _____ (_____) years of the termination of this Agreement. For purposes of this Section, the geographical service area shall be defined as within (_____) miles of [City], [State]. Notwithstanding the foregoing, (i) this Section shall not be construed to limit Executive from engaging in activities on behalf of a multilocational entity to the extent that his duties and responsibilities relate primarily to locations outside of such geographic service area, and (ii) Executive may own up to _____ percent (_____%) of the outstanding stock of public companies without violating this Section.

(b) For a period of _____ (_____) months thereafter, Executive shall not, unless acting pursuant hereto or with the prior written consent of the Board, directly or indirectly, on Executive's own behalf or as a principal, representative or agent of any person, hospital, healthcare facility, health system, or related business, solicit or induce any employee, contractor, or consultant of the Employer or any Affiliate to terminate, reduce, or otherwise alter his/her relationship with the Employer or any Affiliate or to enter into the employment of or a similar relationship with any other hospital, healthcare facility, health system, or related business. Executive shall not engage in any attempt to divert from the Employer or its Affiliates any business in which the Employer or its Affiliates were actively engaged during his employment, or made material plans to engage in during or after his employment. Notwithstanding the foregoing, if Executive is employed by another entity under circumstances that are not otherwise a violation of this Section 6, Executive may employ or solicit contractors or consultants of the Employer or its Affiliates to provide Services to Executive's new employer on a nonexclusive basis.

(c) Executive acknowledges that the restrictions contained in this Section 6 are, in view of the nature of the business of the Employer and its Affiliates, reasonable and necessary to protect the legitimate interests of the Employer and Affiliates and that any violation of any provision of this Section 6 will result in irreparable injury to the Employer and its Affiliates. Executive also acknowledges that in the event of any such violation, the Employer and/or its Affiliates shall be entitled to preliminary and permanent injunctive relief, without the necessity of proving actual damages, and to the equitable accounting of all earnings, profits, and other benefits arising from any such violation, which rights shall be cumulative and in addition to any other rights or remedies to which the Employer and/or its Affiliates may be entitled. Executive agrees that in the event of any such violation, an action may be commenced for any such preliminary and permanent injunctive relief and other equitable relief in any federal or state court of competent jurisdiction. Further, Executive hereby waives, to the fullest extent permitted by law, any objection that Executive may now or hereafter have to such jurisdiction or to the laying of the venue of any such suit, action or proceeding brought in such a court and any claim that such suit, action or proceeding has been brought in an inconvenient forum.

7. **Adequate Consideration.**

The Employer and Executive each agree that the consideration set forth in this Separation Agreement is adequate and sufficient consideration to extinguish any right or obligation that either party may have to the other party pursuant to the Employment Agreement. As such, the Employer and Executive each agree not to commence any arbitration, mediation, claim, or proceeding, or any other form of action in law or equity, against each other, arising out of or related to the execution, performance or termination of Executive's employment and hereby waive all rights to the same.

8. **Releases.**

(a) The Employer, on behalf of itself and its respective officers, directors, agents, executives, representatives, affiliates, successors and assigns, hereby agrees to fully release, discharge and forever hold harmless Executive and his estate, representatives, executors, and heirs from any and all liability or claims (including, but not limited to, claims for damages, punitive damages, costs, or attorneys' fees), whether known or unknown, related to or arising out of the execution or performance of Executive's duties while employed by the Employer, other than intentional wrongful conduct on the part of Executive.

(b) Executive, on behalf of himself and his estate, representatives, executors and heirs, successors, and assigns, hereby agrees to fully release, discharge, and forever hold harmless the Employer and its officers, trustees, agents, executives, representatives, affiliates, successors and assigns from any and all liability or claims (including, but not limited to, claims for damages, punitive damages, costs, or attorneys' fees), whether known or unknown, related to or arising out of the Employment Agreement, the Severance Plan, any action taken by the same related to Executive's employment with the Employer, the execution of this Agreement or the termination of Executive's employment. Said release shall include, but not be limited to, any claim or action that may now or hereafter be asserted by Executive purporting to be violations of any state or federal statutes such as Title VII of the Civil Rights Act of 1964, the Americans with Disabilities Act, the Family and Medical Leave Act, the Age Discrimination in Employment Act of 1967, [applicable state law], federal or state or common law, or the Constitution of any state or of the United States, and Executive hereby expressly waives any and all legal or equitable remedies which may have been available to him thereunder including, but not limited to, any claim for attorneys' fees.

(c) The releases set forth in Sections 8(a) and (b) do not preclude Executive from seeking indemnification from any action arising out of the acts or omissions of Executive while he was the Chief Executive Officer of the Employer.

(d) Executive represents that he has provided the Employer with any and all information that he possesses that he reasonably believes might cause the Employer or any of its Affiliates to incur any civil or criminal liability to the state or federal government and, as such, hereby waives any right he may now or hereafter possess to act as a relator in a qui tam suit against the Employer on behalf of the United States and/or the State of _____ under the False Claims Act or any similar federal or state statute and further agrees never to file any such suit.

(e) In the event that Executive or his estate, representatives, heirs, or executors bring any action or claim for any matter subject to the release set forth in this Section, all payments due to Executive hereunder shall cease, and the benefits provided under this Agreement shall be forfeited.

(f) Notwithstanding the above, if any party violates the terms and conditions of this Agreement, the aggrieved party may pursue an appropriate action at law or equity to enforce this Agreement.

(g) The foregoing releases may never be treated as an admission of liability by either party for any purpose.

9. **Cooperation in Event of Claims or Investigations; Indemnification; Continued Insurance Coverage.**

(a) The parties will fully cooperate with each other in the event that any claims are brought against either or both of them or investigations are instituted by government agencies regarding matters related to the activities of the Employer or Executive while he was employed by the Employer. The Executive specifically agrees to provide testimony and/or participate in strategy sessions with respect to litigation, claims or investigations when requested to do so by the Employer. The Employer shall reimburse Executive for expenses associated with the same.

(b) The Employer will indemnify Executive to the fullest extent permitted by applicable laws and regulations in connection with any claims or investigations arising from his employment by the Employer and in connection with any action undertaken while he was the Chief Executive Officer of or acting at the behest or on behalf of the Employer and within the scope of his employment. This will include advancing the costs of defense incurred by Executive to the extent permitted by the laws of the State of _____, provided that the Employer approves Executive's counsel and Executive is party to any joint defense agreement that the Employer may propose.

(c) The Employer agrees to continue to cover Executive under its director's and officer's and other liability insurance (to the extent permitted by said insurance policy) and to provide a defense to him against all costs, charges, and expenses incurred in connection with any action, suit, or proceeding to which he may be made a party by reasons of his duties as Chief Executive Officer of the Employer or for services requested by the Employer under this Agreement.

## 10. No Representations.

This document constitutes the final, complete, and exclusive statement of the terms of the agreement among all the parties to this Agreement relating to the rights granted by it and the obligations assumed under it. No party has been induced to enter into this Agreement by, nor has any party relied on, any representation or warranty outside those expressly set forth in this Agreement. This Agreement may be supplemented, amended, or modified only by the mutual agreement of the parties, in writing signed by all the parties. If a court or an arbitrator of competent jurisdiction holds any provision of this Agreement to be illegal, unenforceable, or invalid in whole or in part for any reason, the validity and enforceability of the remaining provisions, or portions of them, will not be affected.

## 11. Successors.

All of the terms and provisions contained in this Agreement shall inure to the benefit of and shall be binding upon the parties hereto and their respective heirs, legal representatives, successors, and assigns.

## 12. Severability and Governing Law.

(a) With the exception of Section 8(a) and (b), should any of the provisions in this Agreement be declared or be determined to be illegal or invalid, all remaining parts, terms or provisions shall be valid, and the illegal or invalid part, term, or provision shall be deemed not to be a part of this Agreement.

(b) This Agreement is made and entered into in the State of _____ and shall in all respects be interpreted, enforced and governed under the laws of _____. Venue for resolution of disputes shall be in [county], [state].

## 13. Proper Construction.

(a) The language of all parts of this Agreement shall in all cases be construed as a whole according to its fair meaning, and not strictly for or against any of the parties.

(b) As used in this Agreement, the term "or" shall be deemed to include the term "and/or" and the singular or plural number shall be deemed to include the other whenever the context so indicates or requires.

(c) The paragraph headings used in this Agreement are intended solely for convenience of reference and shall not in any manner amplify, limit, modify, or otherwise be used in the interpretation of any of the provisions hereof.

## 14. Understanding of Consequences.

(a) The parties have been advised by counsel and understand and acknowledge the significance and consequence of the specific intention to release all claims and thereby assume full responsibility for any injuries, damages, losses, or liability that they may hereafter incur.

(b) Executive further certifies that he has read the terms of this Agreement, including the Releases in Section 8, and has had an opportunity to review this Agreement with his attorney, and that he understands its terms and effects. Executive further acknowledges that he is executing this Agreement voluntarily, with a full understanding of its terms and effects, in exchange for consideration which he acknowledges is adequate and satisfactory to him. Executive further represents and warrants that he has been informed that he has up to twenty-one (21) days to review this Agreement before signing it and that he may revoke all parts of this Agreement within twenty-one (21) days of signing it by informing the Employer of such revocation in writing on or before the seventh day. If Executive exercises his option to revoke this Agreement, this Agreement shall be entirely null and void

## 15. Counterparts; Execution.

This Agreement may be executed in one or more counterparts, and by the different parties hereto in separate counterparts, each of which when executed shall be deemed to be an original, but all of which taken together shall constitute one and the same agreement. This Agreement may be executed by facsimile.

IN WITNESS WHEREOF, the parties have caused this Agreement to be executed on the date written below.

**EMPLOYER**

WITNESS: _____ BY: _____

[Name/Title]

DATE: _____

WITNESS: _____

DATE: _____          _____

[Name of Executive]

# EXHIBIT A

## BENEFITS CONTINUED DURING SEVERANCE PERIOD

The following benefits shall be continued during the time that Executive receives severance pay in accordance with Section 2(b) of the Separation Agreement: [Relevant benefits, if any, would be listed here.]

# Common Healthcare Abbreviations and Definitions

*Iowa Hospital Association*

This book would be greatly remiss if it did not comment on the "foreign" language of healthcare. As with many other industries, healthcare has spawned its own lexicon, inhabited by a seemingly unending stream of abbreviations and special jargon—as confusing to board members as it is to the general public. CEOs of healthcare organizations, and others to whom the jargon is a normal part of their daily lives, must remember to communicate with their boards and the public using as little healthcare terminology as possible because it can be intimidating, frustrating, and confusing for the listener. Board members who have become comfortable with the lingo should also remember that same caution.

As a personal example, I remember entering a doctoral program at a major university after being a hospital CEO and merging two hospitals. I was attending a general business faculty meeting and everyone kept referring to the problems they were having with the "OB" courses. I kept thinking to myself, "Why is obstetrics a problem here?" When I asked, I was told that in their setting, "OB" referred to organizational behavior, not obstetrics.

Board members should never hesitate to ask what a term or concept means. They don't deal with the terminology on a daily basis and should not be expected to know the terms. Appendix 7 provides a basic list of common healthcare abbreviations and terms to help board members negotiate their way through this fascinating industry.

*Errol L. Biggs*

# COMMON HEALTHCARE ABBREVIATIONS
# AND DEFINITIONS

Iowa Hospital Association. 2008. "Common Healthcare Abbreviations &
Terminology." See www.ihaonline.org/publications/termsweb.pdf.

**AAHP**     American Association of Health Plans

**AAPCC**     average adjusted per capita cost

**ACHE**     American College of Healthcare Executives

**ADC**     average daily census

**ADS**     alternative delivery systems

**AHA**     American Hospital Association or American Heart Association

**AHRQ**     Agency for Health Care Research and Quality

**ALOS**     average length of stay

**AMA**     against medical advice or American Medical Association

**ANA**     American Nurses Association

**ANP**     advanced nurse practitioner

**ART**     accredited record technician

**ASC**     ambulatory surgery center

**BBA**     Balanced Budget Act of 1997

**BBRA**     Balanced Budget Relief Act of 1999

**BMR**     basal metabolism rate

**BP**     blood pressure

**CAH**     critical access hospital

**CAM**     complementary and alternative medicine

**CAT**     computerized axial tomography

**CBC**     complete blood count

**CCU**     cardiac care unit

**CDC**     Centers for Disease Control

**CIO**     chief information officer

| CMI | case mix index |
| CMS | Centers for Medicare & Medicaid Services |
| CNM | certified nurse midwife |
| CNS | central nervous system |
| CON | certificate of need |
| CPR | cardiopulmonary resuscitation |
| CQI | continuous quality improvement |
| CRNA | certified registered nurse anesthetist |
| CVA | cerebrovascular accident, a stroke |
| CVI | cerebrovascular insufficiency |
| D&C | dilatation and curettage |
| DC | doctor of chiropractic |
| DDS | doctor of dental surgery |
| DHHS | Department of Health and Human Services (federal) |
| DME | durable medical equipment |
| DNR | do not resuscitate, also do not report |
| DO | doctor of osteopathy (osteopathic physician) |
| DPM | doctor of podiatric medicine |
| DRG | diagnosis related group |
| DSH | disproportionate share hospital |
| DVM | doctor of veterinary medicine |
| ECF | extended care facility |
| EEG | electroencephalogram |
| EKG | electrocardiogram |
| EMG | electromyogram |
| EMR | electronic medical record |
| EMS | emergency medical services |
| EMT | emergency medical technician |
| ENT | ear, nose and throat |

| | |
|---|---|
| **FACHE** | Fellow of the American College of Healthcare Executives |
| **FFS** | fee for service |
| **FMG** | foreign medical graduate |
| **FQHC** | federally qualified health center |
| **FTE** | full-time equivalent |
| **GI** | gastrointestinal |
| **GP** | general practitioner |
| **GU** | genitourinary |
| **IOM** | Institute of Medicine |
| **HHS** | Health and Human Services (federal) |
| **IDS** | integrated delivery system |
| **IPA** | independent practice association |
| **IV** | intravenous |
| **LOS** | length of stay |
| **LTC** | long-term care |
| **MCO** | managed care organization |
| **MD** | medical doctor (allopathic physican) |
| **MOB** | medical office building |
| **MRI** | magnetic resonance imaging |
| **MSA** | metropolitan statistical area |
| **MSO** | management service organization |
| **ND** | doctor of naturopathic medicine or nursing doctorate |
| **OB-GYN** | obstetrics and gynecology |
| **OD** | doctor of optometry |
| **OSHA** | Occupational Safety and Health Administration |
| **PA** | physician's assistant |
| **PCN** | primary care network |
| **PET** | positron emission tomography |
| **PHO** | physician hospital organization |

| | |
|---|---|
| **POS** | point of service |
| **PPO** | preferred provider organization |
| **PPS** | prospective payment system |
| **PCP** | primary care physician |
| **PSA** | prostate specific antigen |
| **PSO** | provider sponsored organization |
| **QA** | quality assurance |
| **QI** | quality improvement |
| **RBC** | red blood count |
| **RBRVS** | resource-based relative value scale |
| **SARS** | severe acute respiratory syndrome |
| **SIDS** | sudden infant death syndrome |
| **SNF** | skilled nursing facility |
| **SPECT** | single photon emission computerized tomography |
| **Stark (#)** | Physician referral laws; part of OBRA '89 ("Stark I") and '93 ("Stark II") |
| **Stat** | immediately |
| **T&A** | tonsillectomy and adenoidectomy |
| **Temp** | temperature |
| **TQM** | total quality management |
| **UR** | utilization review |
| **WBC** | white blood count |

## HEALTHCARE DEFINITIONS

**ACCOUNTABLE CARE ORGANIZATIONS (ACOs)** – Healthcare organizations that take accountability for both cost and quality of the care they provide to defined populations, and produce performance data on outcomes. These could include physician practices, hospitals and other entities. The ACO concept was created in H.R. 4872 (the Healthcare Education Reconciliation Act of 2010). By January 1, 2012, at the latest, HHS will establish a Medicare shared savings program that promotes accountability for a patient population.

**ACUITY** – degree or severity of illness

**ACQUIRED IMMUNE DEFICIENCY SYNDROME (AIDS)** – A fatal, incurable disease caused by a virus that can destroy the body's ability to fight off illness, resulting in recurrent opportunistic infections or secondary diseases afflicting multiple body systems.

**ACUTE CARE HOSPITAL** – Typically a community hospital that has services designed to meet the needs of patients who require short-term care for a period of less than 30 days.

**ADVANCE DIRECTIVE** – Written instructions recognized under law relating to the provision of healthcare when an individual is incapacitated. An advance directive takes two forms: living wills and durable power of attorney for healthcare.

**ALLOWABLE CHARGE** – Term used by Medicare (or other third party) to define the amount of a bill it will consider for payment.

**ALTERNATE DELIVERY SYSTEMS** – Health services provided in other than an inpatient, acute care hospital, such as skilled and nursing facilities, hospice programs, and home healthcare.

**AMBULATORY CARE** – Medical care provided on an outpatient basis.

**AMBULATORY PAYMENT CLASSIFICATION (APC)** –The method CMS uses to classify outpatient services and procedures that are comparable clinically and in terms of resource use; serves as the basis of the Medicare Outpatient PPS.

**ANCILLARY** – A term used to describe services that relate to a patient's care such as lab work, x-ray, and anesthesia.

**AVERAGE ADJUSTED PER CAPITA COST (AAPCC)** – The methodology used to develop the premium rate paid to HMOs by the federal government for Medicare recipients in a given geographic region based on historical service costs.

**AVERAGE DAILY CENSUS (ADC)** – The average number of hospital inpatients per day. The ADC is calculated by dividing the total number of patient days during a given period by the number of calendar days in that period.

**AVERAGE LENGTH OF STAY (ALOS)** – The average number of days in a given time period that each patient remains in the hospital. ALOS varies by type of admission, age, and sex. To calculate ALOS, divide the total number of bed days by the number of discharges for a specified period.

**BENCHMARKING** – A process which identifies best practices and performance standards, to create normative or comparative standards (benchmark) as a measurement tool. By comparing an organization against a national or regional benchmark, providers are able to establish measurable goals as part of the strategic planning and Total Quality Management (TQM) processes.

**BOARD CERTIFIED** – Describes a physician who is certified as a specialist in her area of practice. To achieve board certification, a physician must meet specific standards of knowledge and clinical skills within a specific field or specialty. Usually, this means completion of a supervised program of certified clinical residency and the physician passing both an oral and written examination given by a medical specialty group.

**BOARD ELIGIBLE** – Describes a physician who has graduated from a board-approved medical school, completed an accredited training program, practiced for a specified length of time, and is eligible to take a specialty board examination within a specific amount of time.

**CAPITAL EXPENSE** – An expenditure that benefits more than one accounting period, such as the cost to acquire long-term assets. Capital investment decisions typically involve large sums of money for long periods of time and have a major impact on the future services provided by an organization.

**CAPITALIZE** – To record an expenditure that may benefit a future period as an asset rather than as an expense of the period of its occurrence. For example, research and development costs.

**CAPITATION** – Method of payment for health services in which the insurer pays providers a fixed amount for each person served regardless of the type and number of services used.

**CARDIAC CATHETERIZATION** – A procedure used to diagnose disorders of the heart, lungs, and great vessels.

**CASE MANAGEMENT** – A managed care technique in which a patient with a serious medical condition is assigned an individual who arranges for cost-effective treatment, often outside a hospital.

**CAT (COMPUTERIZED AXIAL TOMOGRAPHY)** – Diagnostic equipment which produces cross-sectional images of the head and/or body.

**CENSUS** – The number of inpatients who receive hospital care each day, excluding newborns.

**CENTERS FOR MEDICARE & MEDICAID SERVICES (CMS)** – The federal agency responsible for administering Medicare, Medicaid, and the State Children's Health Insurance Program (SCHIP).

**CHEMOTHERAPY** – In the treatment of disease, the application of chemical reagents which have a specific and toxic effect upon the disease-causing microorganism.

**CLOSED PANEL** – A managed care plan that contracts with or employs physicians on an exclusive basis for services and does not allow those physicians to see patients from other managed care organizations. Staff model HMOs are examples of closed-panel managed care plans.

**CODE BLUE** – Indicates an emergency situation has occurred and mobilizes staff to respond.

**COMMUNITY RATING** – A method of calculating health insurance premiums in which the health status and plan use of employer groups and individuals are combined and a single rate is paid by all groups and individuals.

**CONCURRENT REVIEW** – A managed care technique in which a representative of a managed care firm continuously reviews the charts of hospitalized patients to determine whether they are staying too long and if the course of treatment is appropriate.

**CONSOLIDATED OMNIBUS BUDGET RECONCILIATION ACT (COBRA)** – Federal law that requires employers with more than 20 employees to extend group health insurance coverage for at least 18 months after employees leave their jobs. Employees must pay 100 percent of the premium.

**CONSUMER PRICE INDEX, MEDICAL CARE COMPONENT** – An inflationary measure encompassing the cost of all purchased healthcare services.

**COST-SHIFTING** – A phenomenon in which providers are inadequately reimbursed for their costs by some payers and subsequently raise their prices to other payers in an effort to recoup costs. Low reimbursement rates from government healthcare programs often cause providers to raise prices for medical care to private insurance carriers.

**CREDENTIALING AND PRIVILEGING** – Process by which hospitals determine the scope of practice of practitioners providing services in the hospital; criteria for granting privileges or credentialing are determined by the hospital and include individual character, competence, training, experience, and judgment.

**CRITICAL ACCESS HOSPITAL (CAH)** – Part of the Medicare Rural Hospital Flexibility Program created by BBA97. A critical access hospital is a limited service, small rural hospital that receives cost-based reimbursement for inpatient and outpatient care.

**DIAGNOSIS-RELATED GROUP (DRG)** – A resource classification system that serves as the basis of the method for reimbursing hospitals based on the medical diagnosis for each patient. Hospitals receive a set payment amount determined in advance based on the length of time patients with a given diagnosis are likely to stay in the hospital. Also used as the basis of the Medicare inpatient prospective payment system (PPS).

**DIRECT CONTRACTING** – Refers to a direct contractual arrangement between an employer and a provider or provider organization, for the provision of healthcare services. The two parties may negotiate rates for services in a variety of ways, such as discounted charges, per diem rates, or DRGs. Direct contracts may include use of third party administrators for claims processing, utilization management, or other administrative functions. Direct contracting is often used as a cost containment strategy since fewer costs are incurred by a "middleman" insurance company.

**DURABLE POWER OF ATTORNEY FOR HEALTHCARE** – Allows an individual to designate in advance another person to act on his behalf if he is unable to make a decision to accept, maintain, discontinue, or refuse any healthcare services.

**EXCLUSIVE PROVIDER ORGANIZATION (EPO)** – A healthcare payment and delivery arrangement in which members must obtain all their care from doctors and hospitals within an established network. If members go outside, benefits are not payable.

**FORMULARY** – The list of prescription medications that may be dispensed by participating pharmacies without health plan authorization. The formulary is selected based on effectiveness of the drug as well as its cost. The physician is requested or required to use only formulary drugs unless there is a valid medical reason to use a nonformulary drug. Formularies may be open or closed. Closed formularies are restricted by the number and type of drugs included in the list.

**FREESTANDING AMBULATORY SURGERY CENTER** – A medical facility which provides surgical treatment on an outpatient basis only.

**FULL-TIME EQUIVALENT PERSONNEL (FTES)** – Refers to hospital employees; total FTE personnel is calculated by dividing the hospital's total number of paid hours by 2080, the number of annual paid hours for one full-time employee.

**GATEKEEPER** – Term used to describe the coordination role of the primary care provider (PCP) who manages various components of a member's medical treatment, including all referrals for specialty care, ancillary services, durable medical equipment, and hospital services. The gatekeeper model is a popular cost-control component of many managed care plans because it requires a subscriber to first see their PCP and receive the PCP's approval before going to a specialist about a given medical condition (except for emergencies).

**HEALTH AND HUMAN SERVICES (HHS)** – The US Department of Health and Human Services. formerly Department of Health, Education, and Welfare.

**HEALTH MAINTENANCE ORGANIZATION (HMO)** – A healthcare payment and delivery system involving networks of doctors and hospitals. Members must receive all their care from providers within the network.

- *Staff Model HMO.* Physicians are on the staff of the HMO and are usually paid a salary.

- *Group Model HMO.* The HMO rents the services of the physicians in a separate group practice and pays the group a per-patient rate.

- *Network Model HMO.* The HMO contracts with two or more independent physician group practices to provide services and pays a fixed monthly fee per patient.

**HOSPICE** – An organization that provides medical care and support services (such as pain and symptom management, counseling, and bereavement services) to terminally ill patients and their families; may be a freestanding facility, a unit of a hospital or other institution, or a separate program of a hospital, agency, or institution.

**HOSPITALISTS** – A physician whose practice is caring for patients while in the hospital. A primary care physician (PCP) turns their patients over to a hospitalist, who becomes the physician of record, provides and directs the care of the patient while the patient is hospitalized, and returns the patient to the PCP at the time of hospital discharge.

**HOSPITAL MARKET BASKET INDEX (HMBI)** – An inflationary measure of the cost of goods and services purchased by hospitals.

**HOSPITAL PREAUTHORIZATION** – A managed care technique in which the insured obtains permission from a managed care organization before entering the hospital for nonemergency care.

**INDEPENDENT PRACTICE ASSOCIATION (IPA)** – A group of independent physicians who have formed an association as a separate legal entity for contracting purposes. IPA physician providers retain their individual practices, work in separate offices, continue to see their non-managed care patients, and have the option to contract directly with managed care plans. A key advantage of the IPA arrangement is that it helps its members achieve some of the negotiating leverage of a large physician group practice with some degree of flexibility for each provider. Also referred to as independent physician association.

**INTEGRATED CARE** – A comprehensive spectrum of health services, from prevention through long-term care, provided via a single administrative entity and coordinated by a primary care "gatekeeper."

**INTEGRATED DELIVERY NETWORKS OR SYSTEM (IDN OR IDS)** – An entity (corporation, partnership, association, or other legal entity) that enters into arrangements with managed care organizations; employs or has contracts with providers; and agrees to provide or arrange for the provision of healthcare services to members covered by the managed care plan.

**THE JOINT COMMISSION** – The organization that evaluates and monitors the quality of care provided in hospitals.

**LENGTH OF STAY (LOS)** – The period of hospitalization as measured in days billed; average length of stay is determined by discharge days divided by discharges.

**LIVING WILL** – Document generated by a person for the purpose of providing guidance about the medical care to be provided if the person is unable to articulate those decisions (see advance directive).

**LONG-TERM CARE** – A continuum of maintenance, custodial, and health services to the chronically ill, disabled, or mentally handicapped.

**MAGNETIC RESONANCE IMAGING (MRI)** – A noninvasive diagnostic technique used to create images of body tissue and monitor body chemistry; uses radio and magnetic waves instead of radiation.

**MANAGED CARE** – A term that applies to the integration of healthcare delivery and financing. It includes arrangements with providers to supply healthcare services to members, criteria for the selection of healthcare providers, significant financial incentives for members to use providers in the plan, and formal programs to monitor the amount of care and quality of services. A healthcare organization, such as a health maintenance organization, that "manages" or controls what it spends on healthcare by closely monitoring how doctors and other medical professionals treat patients.

**MANAGEMENT SERVICE ORGANIZATION (MSO)** – An entity that provides practice management and other operational services to physicians, which can include facilitating managed care contracting.

**MANDATED BENEFITS** – Certain services or benefits, such as prenatal care, mammographic screening, and care for newborns, that states require insurers to include in health insurance policies. Sometimes called state mandates.

**MEDICAID** – A federal public assistance program enacted into law on January 1, 1966, under Title XIX of the Social Security Act, to provide medical benefits to eligible low-income persons needing healthcare regardless of age. The program is administered and operated by the states which receive federal matching funds to cover the costs of the program. States are required to include certain minimal services as mandated by the federal government but may include any additional services at their own expense.

**MEDICAL LOSS RATIO** – The ratio between the cost to deliver medical care and the amount of money that a plan receives. Insurance companies often have a medical loss ratio of 92 percent or more; tightly managed HMOs may have medical loss ratios of 75 to 85 percent, although the overhead (or administrative cost ratio) is concomitantly higher. The medical loss ratio is dependent on the amount of money brought in, as well as the cost of delivering care; thus, if the rates are too low, the ratio may be high, even though the actual cost of delivering care is not out of line.

**MEDICARE GEOGRAPHIC CLASSIFICATION REVIEW BOARD** – Five-person board, established by Congress in 1990, to review hospital requests for geographic reclassification for Medicare prospective payment system (PPS) purposes; to be reclassified, hospitals generally must be located in an adjacent county and pay wages equal to at least 85 percent of those paid by hospitals in the area for which reclassification is being requested.

**MEDICARE-SUPPLEMENT POLICY** – A type of health insurance policy that provides benefits for services Medicare does not cover.

**MEDIGAP INSURANCE** – A supplemental health insurance policy in which a Medicare beneficiary pays a monthly premium to cover the cost of health benefits that Medicare does not cover.

**MedPAC** – Medicare Payment Advisory Commission created by Congress in 1997 for the purpose of making recommendations regarding the Medicare program to Congress. This commission replaces the Physician Payment Review Commission (PPRC) and the Prospective Payment Assessment Commission (ProPAC).

**MORBIDITY** – Incidence and severity of illness and accidents in a well defined class or classes of individuals.

**MORTALITY** – Incidence of death in a well defined class or classes of individuals.

**MULTIHOSPITAL SYSTEM** – Two or more hospitals owned, leased, contract managed, or sponsored by a central organization; they can be either not-for-profit or investor-owned.

**NEONATAL** – The part of an infant's life from the hour of birth through the first 27 days, 23 hours and 59 minutes; the infant is referred to as newborn throughout this period.

**NOSOCOMIAL INFECTION** – Infection acquired in a hospital.

**NUCLEAR MEDICINE** – The use of radioisotopes to study and treat disease, especially in the diagnostic area.

**NURSE PRACTITIONER (NP)** – A licensed nurse who has completed a nurse practitioner program at the master's or certificate level and is trained in providing primary care services. NPs are qualified to conduct expanded healthcare evaluations and decision making regarding patient care, including diagnosis, treatment, and prescriptions, sometimes under a physician's supervision. They generally provide services at a lower cost than PCPs. NPs may also be trained in medical specialties, such as pediatrics, geriatrics, and midwifery. Legal regulations in some states prevent NPs from qualifying for direct Medicare and Medicaid reimbursement, writing prescriptions, and admitting patients to hospitals. Also called advance practice nurse (APN).

**NURSING LEVELS OF EDUCATION** – The levels of education established for nursing are:

- Licensed practical nurse (LPN) requires one year of formal training at a vocational or technical school;

- Diploma (RN) requires two to three years of education at a hospital school of nursing;

- Associate's degree (ADN) requires two years of education at a community college or university;

- Baccalaureate degree (BSN) requires four academic years of education at a college or university.

- Master's degree (MS or MSN) requires completion of at least one year of prescribed study beyond the baccalaureate degree.

**OPEN PANEL** – Allows for any willing provider to contract with an HMO providing the provider meets all the requirements set forth by the HMO.

**OPERATING MARGIN** – Margin of net patient care revenues in excess of operating expenses.

**OUT-OF-NETWORK SERVICES** – Healthcare services received by a plan member from a noncontracted provider. Reimbursement is usually lower when a member goes out of network. Other financial penalties may apply for out-of-network services.

**OUTCOMES** – The end result of medical care, as indicated by recovery, disability, functional status, mortality, morbidity, or patient satisfaction.

**OUTCOMES MEASUREMENT** – The process of systematically tracking a patient's clinical treatment and responses to that treatment using generally accepted outcomes measures or quality indicators, such as mortality, morbidity, disability, functional status, recovery, and patient satisfaction. Such measures are considered by many healthcare researchers as the only valid way to determine the effectiveness of medical care.

**OUTPATIENT CARE** – Treatment provided to a patient who is not confined in a healthcare facility. Outpatient care includes services that do not require an overnight stay, such as emergency treatment, same-day surgery, outpatient diagnostic tests, and physician office visits. Also referred to as ambulatory care.

**PATIENT DAYS** – Refers to each calendar day of care provided to a hospital inpatient under the terms of the patient's health plan, excluding the day of discharge. "Patient days" is a measure of institutional use and is usually stated as the accumulated total number of inpatients (excluding newborns) each day for a given reporting period, tallied at a specified time (like midnight) per 1,000 use rate, or patient days/1,000. Patient days are calculated by multiplying admissions by average length of stay (ALOS).

**PATIENT SATISFACTION SURVEY** – Questionnaire used to solicit the perceptions of plan enrollees/patients regarding how a health plan meets their medical needs and how the delivery of care is handled (e.g., waiting time, access to treatments).

**PEER REVIEW** – An evaluation of the appropriateness, effectiveness, and efficiency of medical services ordered or performed by practicing physicians or professionals by other practicing physicians or clinical professionals. A peer review focuses on the quality of services that are performed by all health personnel involved in the delivery of the care under review and how appropriate the services are to meet the patients' needs.

**PHYSICIAN HOSPITAL ORGANIZATION (PHO)** – A type of integrated delivery system that links hospitals and a group of physicians for the purpose of contracting directly with employers and managed care organizations. A PHO is a legal entity which allows physicians to continue to own their own practices and to see patients under the terms of a professional services agreement. This type of arrangement offers the opportunity to better market the services of both physicians and hospitals as a unified response to managed care.

**PHYSICIAN'S ASSISTANT (PA)** – A specially trained and licensed allied health professional, who performs certain medical procedures previously reserved for the physician. PAs must practice under the supervision of a physician.

**POINT OF SERVICE** – Members in a point of service HMO or PPO can go outside the network for care, but their copay and deductible will be more than if they had used providers who are part of the HMO, PPO, or health plan.

**POINT-OF-SERVICE PLAN (POS)** – A type of managed care plan that allows patients to choose how to receive services at the point when the services are needed. They may use "out of network providers" for an additional fee. Also called open-ended HMO, swing-out HMO, self-referral option, or multiple option plan.

**POSITRON EMISSION TOMOGRAPHY (PET)** – An imaging, technique which tracks metabolism and responses to therapy. Used in cardiology, neurology, and oncology; particularly effective in evaluating brain and nervous system disorders

**PRACTICE GUIDELINES** – Formal procedures and techniques for the treatment of specific medical conditions that assist physicians in achieving optimal results. Practice guidelines are developed by medical societies and medical research organizations, such as the American Medical Association (AMA) and the Agency for Health Care Policy and Research (AHCPR), as well as many HMOs, insurers, and business coalitions. Practice guidelines serve as educational support for physicians and as quality assurance and accountability measures for managed care plans.

**PREADMISSION CERTIFICATION** – Process in which a healthcare professional evaluates an attending physician's request for a patient's admission to a hospital by using established medical criteria.

**PREFERRED PROVIDER ORGANIZATION (PPO)** – A plan that contracts with independent providers at a discount for services. Generally, the PPO's network of providers is limited in size. Patients usually have free choice to select other providers but are given strong financial incentives to select one of the designated preferred providers. Unlike an HMO, a PPO is not a prepaid plan but does use some utilization management techniques. PPO arrangements can be either insured or self-funded. An insurer sponsored PPO combines a large network of providers, utilization management programs, administrative services, and healthcare insurance. A self-funded PPO generally excludes administrative and insurance services from the plan package. However, employers can purchase these services separately.

**PRIMARY CARE NETWORK (PCN)** – A group of primary care physicians (PCP) who share the risk of providing care to members of a managed care plan. The PCP in a primary care network is accountable for the total healthcare services of a plan member, including referrals to specialists, supervision of the specialists' care, and hospitalization. Participating PCPs' services are covered by a monthly capitation payment to the PCN.

**PROSPECTIVE PAYMENT SYSTEM (PPS)** – Also called prospective pricing; a payment method in which the payment a hospital will receive for patient treatment is set up in advance; hospitals keep the difference if they incur costs less than the fixed price in treating the patient and they absorb any loss if their costs exceed the fixed price.

**PROVIDER SPONSORED ORGANIZATION (PSO)** – Public or private entities established or organized and operated by a health provider or a group of affiliated healthcare providers that provide a substantial proportion of services under the Medicare+Choice contract and share substantial financial risk.

**QUALITY ASSURANCE** – Term that describes attempts by managed care organizations to measure and monitor the quality of care delivered.

**QUALITY IMPROVEMENT ORGANIZATION (QIO)** – Federally funded physician organizations, under contract to the Department of Health and Human Services, that review quality of care and determine whether services are necessary and payment should be made for care provided under the Medicare and Medicaid programs.

**REASONABLE AND CUSTOMARY CHARGE** – Charge for healthcare which is consistent with the going rate or charge in a certain geographical area for identical or similar services; also referred to as "customary, prevailing, and reasonable."

**RELATIVE VALUE SCALE (RVS)** – A pricing system for physicians' services which assigns relative values to procedures based on a defined standard unit of measure, as defined in the current procedural terminology (CPT). RVS units are based on median charges by physicians. Physicians often use the RVS system as a guide in establishing fee schedules. This system is rapidly being replaced by RBRVS -based payment systems.

**RESOURCE BASED RELATIVE VALUE SCALE (RBRVS)** – A fee schedule used as the basis of the physician reimbursement system by Medicare. The RBRVS assigns relative values to each CPT code for services on the basis of the resources related to the procedure rather than simply on the basis of historical trends.

**RESTRICTED FUNDS** – Includes all hospital resources that are restricted to particular purposes by donors and other external authorities; the resources of these funds are not currently available for the financing of general operating activities but may be so used in the future when certain conditions and requirements are met; there are three types of restricted funds: (1) specific purpose, (2) plant replacement and expansion, and (3) endowment.

**SEAMLESS CARE** – The experience by patients of smooth and easy movement from one aspect of comprehensive healthcare to another, notable for the absence of red tape.

**SINGLE PAYER SYSTEM** – A financing system, such as Canada's, in which a single entity (usually the government) pays for all covered healthcare services.

**SKILLED NURSING FACILITY (SNF)** – A facility, either freestanding or part of a hospital, that accepts patients in need of rehabilitation and medical care. To qualify for Medicare coverage, SNFs must be certified by Medicare and meet specific qualifications, including 24-hour nursing coverage and availability of physical, occupational, and speech therapies.

**SURGICENTER** – A healthcare facility that is physically separate from a hospital and provides prescheduled surgical services on an outpatient basis, generally at a lower cost than inpatient hospital care. Also called a free-standing outpatient surgery center.

**SWING BEDS** – Acute care hospital beds that can also be used for long-term care, depending on the needs of the patient and the community; only those hospitals with fewer than 100 beds and located in a rural community, where long-term care may be inaccessible, are eligible to have swing beds.

**TEACHING HOSPITALS** – Hospitals that have an accredited medical residency training program and are typically affiliated with a medical school.

**TERTIARY CARE** – Refers to highly technical services for the patient who is in imminent danger of major disability or death.

**THIRD-PARTY ADMINISTRATION (TPA)** – Administration of a group insurance plan by some person or firm other than the insurer or the policyholder.

**TRIAGE** – Evaluation of patient conditions for urgency and seriousness and the establishment of a priority list in order to direct care and ensure the efficient use of medical and nursing staff and facilities.

**UB-92** – The uniform billing claim form developed by CMS and used by hospitals across the nation to bill for services. Some managed care plans demand more detail than is available on the UB-92, requiring the hospitals to send additional itemized billing information.

**ULTRASOUND** – Refers to sound that has different velocities in tissues which differ in density and elasticity from others; this property permits outlining the shape of various tissues and organs in the body.

**URGENT CARE** – Care for injury, illness, or another type of condition (usually not life threatening) which should be treated within 24 hours. Also refers to after-hours care, and to a health plan's classification of hospital admissions as urgent, semi-urgent, or elective.

**USUAL, CUSTOMARY, AND REASONABLE (UCR)** – Amounts charged by healthcare providers that are consistent with charges from similar providers for the same or nearly the same services in a given area.

**UTILIZATION REVIEW** – An evaluation of the care and services that patients receive which is based on pre-established criteria and standards.

**WRAPAROUND PLAN** – Refers to insurance or health plan coverage for copays or deductibles that are not covered under a member's base plan. This is often used for Medicare.

# Index

responsibility for, 5

Community health committees, 13

Community health needs assessment, 13, 126, 127–128

Community health status, 125–128; indicators of, 127; measurement of, 126

Community relations, 119–130; effect of stakeholders on, 119–125; with governing board, 17, 142

Compensation: for board directors, 36–37, 38–39; for CEOs, 70, 88; pros and cons of, 38–39; quality improvement performance-based, 86

Competition, from hospitals' medical staff, 6

Complementary and alternative medicine (CAM), 131–140; terminology of, 134–140

Computerized provider order entry (CPOE) systems, 98

Confidentiality, 16, 17; of peer review, 81

Conflict of interest, 8, 15–16, 39, 56–58

Conflict-of-interest policies, 64; disclosure statement for, 147–150; sample of, 143–146

Congestive heart failure treatment, quality standards for, 84–85

Consolidation, 6

Consultants, board members as, 16

Consumer perception, awareness, and satisfaction surveys, 126–127

Continuing education programs, for board members, 5, 7, 60, 141

Core measures, 84–85

Corporate compliance programs, 9

Corporate Director Forum, 22

Corporate Library, 22–23

Corporate opportunity, 8

Corporate social responsibility, 123–129; neglect of, 125–126; stakeholders' perception of, 123–125

County commissioners, 62–63

County hospitals, governing boards of: directors of, 62–63; physician members of, 60; selection of members, 52

Credentialing, 80, 82, 88, 90

Crisis management, 71

Criticism, avoidance of, 15

*Crossing the Quality Chasm* (Institute of Medicine), 83

Current assets, 104, 107

Current liabilities, 104

## D

*Darling* v. *Charleston Community Memorial Hospital,* 80

Dartmouth Institute of Health Policy and Clinical Practice, 95

Dashboards, 4, 28, 88

Days cash on hand, 110

Days in accounts receivable, 111–112

Debt to capitalization, 113–114

Decision making, by physicians, 59

Deep breathing exercises, 132

Defendants, healthcare officers and directors as, 8–9

Definitions, of healthcare. *See* Terminology, of healthcare

Delegation, by governing board members, 71

Demographic data analysis, in community health status assessment, 127

Directives, implementation of, 72

Directors, of governing boards. *See* Board chairs (directors)

Directors and officers (D&O) insurance, 9

Disclosure statements, 147–150

Disruptive/dysfunctional behavior, of board members, 14–15, 36, 47–49

District hospitals: board membership selection for, 52; physician board members of, 60

Duty of care, 7, 13

Duty of loyalty, 8, 13, 56

Duty of obedience, 8–9, 13

## E

EBITDA coverage ratio, 114

EBITDA margin, 112

Educational opportunities. *See also* Continuing education programs: for governing board members, 73

Emergency room physicians, exclusion from board membership, 57

Employment contracts, of CEOs, 68–69; sample of, 157–168

Equipment, accounting age estimation for,

of, 127

Health Research and Educational Trust, 29

Heart angioplasty, quality standards for, 97, 98

Heart attack treatment, quality standards for, 84–85

Heart bypass surgery, quality standards for, 97, 98

Hippocratic Oath, 83

Hospital-associated conditions, 83, 88–89

Hospitalists, exclusion from board membership, 57

Hospital Standardized Mortality Rates, 100

**I**

Illinois, business coalitions on health in, 93

Illness, definition of, 138

Indemnification privileges, 39

Indiana, business coalitions on health in, 93

Inova Health System, 32–33

Institute for Healthcare Improvement, 82, 88, 100; 5 Million Lives Campaign of, 83–84

Institute of Medicine: *Crossing the Quality Chasm* report of, 83; *To Err Is Human* report of, 83, 96

Integrative healthcare, 131

Intellectual ability, age-related changes in, 35

Intensivists, exclusion from board membership, 57

Intermountain Health Care, Salt Lake City, Utah, 63

Internal Revenue Service (IRS) Form 990, 11, 37, 55–56

Investment income, 105

**J**

Jargon, in healthcare, 73. *See also* Abbreviations, in health care; Acronyms, in healthcare

Jessee, William, 62

Job descriptions, 141; of board chairs, 19–20; of board members, 5, 13, 18–22, 21–22, 70; lack of, 70; reviews of, 64; of vice chairs, 20–21

Job termination, of CEOs, 69

Joint Commission, 42, 100; accreditation process of, 90–92; overview of, 89–92;

Standards Interpretation Group of, 91

Juran Institute, 95–96

**K**

Kaiser, Leland, 5

Kansas, business coalitions on health in, 93

**L**

Leapfrog Group, 95, 96–99, 100; impact of, 97–99

Leapfrog Hospital Survey, 97–99

Legal duties, of governing boards: duty of care, 7, 13; duty of loyalty, 8, 13, 56; duty of obedience, 8–9, 13

Liabilities: of board members, 7; financial, 104, 105

Liquidity ratios, 109, 110–112

Long-term assets, 104, 107

Long-term liabilities, 104

Louisiana, business coalition on health in, 93

Loyalty, duty of, 8, 13, 56

**M**

Maine: business coalitions on health in, 93; Leapfrog Hospital Survey of, 98–99

Malpractice insurance, 84

Management: board members' involvement in, 70–71; versus governance, 2, 16, 18, 70–71

Management information, 16; versus governance information, 71, 73

Management plans, 69–70

Management skills, of physician board members, 59

Manuals, 65

Marshall, Donna, 92–100

Maryland, business coalitions on health in, 93

Massage therapy, 132, 133

McKinsey surveys, of corporate social responsibility, 125–126

Medicaid, quality assurance and, 81

Medicaid reimbursement, effect of readmission rate on, 89

Medical directors: exclusion from board membership, 57; importance of, 3

Medical errors: implication for reimbursement, 99; medication-related, 83, 88, 98; as mortality cause, 96

Medical staff: credentialing of, 80, 82, 88, 90; representation on governing boards, 58

Medical staff presidents, 54, 56, 58

Medical technology, implication for strategic planning, 6

Medicare: core measures of, 84–85; as patient satisfaction data source, 85; quality assurance and, 81, 84–85

Medicare reimbursement, "never events"-related reduction in, 88–89

Medication errors, 83, 88, 98

Meditation, 132, 133; definition of, 138

Meetings: agendas of, 18, 28; attendance at, 14, 64; board chairs' presiding over, 17; board members' domination of, 15; efficiency and effectiveness of, 27; frequency of, 26–27; governance information for, 27–28; minutes of, 28; positive contributions to, 14–15; preparation for, 14; time limits on, 2

Memorial Hermann Healthcare System, Houston, Texas, 62

Memory, "corporate," 36

Mentors: board chairs as, 18; board members as, 16

Michigan, business coalitions on health in, 93

Midwest Business Group on Health, 95–96

Minnesota, business coalitions on health in, 93

Mission statements, 2–3; board members' agreement with, 14; board members' commitment to, 54; of business coalitions for health, 95

Missouri, business coalitions on health in, 93

Mobile Infirmary Medical Center, Mobile, Alabama, 62

Montana, business coalitions on health in, 93

Morath, Julie, 61

Morbidity data analysis, in community health status assessments, 127

Mortality, medical errors-related, 96

Mortality data analysis, in community health status assessments, 127

Mortality rate: Hospital Standardized Mortality Rates, 100; quality standards for, 97

Music therapy, 133

**N**

NASDAQ stock exchange, 29

National Association of Corporate Directors, 5–6, 23; surveys conducted by, 26–27, 32, 35, 36

National Business Coalition on Health, 92–94

National Center for Complementary and Alternative Medicine, 131

National Institutes for Health, National Center for Complementary and Alternative Medicine of, 131

National Quality Forum, 100

Net assets, 104, 105

Net patient revenues, 105

Nevada, business coalitions on health in, 92, 93

Nevada Health Care Coalition, 92

"Never events," 88–89

New Jersey, business coalition on health in, 93

New Mexico, CEO turnover rate in, 74

New services, in community healthcare, 126–127

New York State, business coalitions on health in, 93

New York Stock Exchange, 29, 42

Nonprofit healthcare organizations, tax-exempt status of, 4

North Carolina, business coalitions on health in, 93

Nurses, involvement in quality improvement, 85

**O**

Oakwood Healthcare System, Dearborn, Michigan, 63

Obedience, duty of, 8–9, 13

Objectives: board members' commitment to, 54; of CEOs, 69; financial, 103; of governing boards, 18; stakeholder-related, 124

Objectivity, of board members, 54, 60

Office of Personnel Management, 97

Ohio, business coalitions on health in, 93

Older adults, cognitive function in, 35

Operating expenses, 105–106

Operating margin, 112–113

Operating revenue, 106

Operational guidelines, for governing boards, 25–50; age limits, 35–36; annual retreat, 37, 39–41; disruptive or inattentive board members, 47–49; executive sessions, 29; frequency of board meetings, 26–27; governance information, 27–28; optimum board size, 25–26; payment for directors, 36–37, 38–39; selection of board chairs, 29–31; self-assessments, 42–47; term limits, 31–35

Opportunities: corporate, 8; identification of, 17

Oregon: business coalitions on health in, 93; CEO turnover rate in, 74

Orientation programs, for new board members, 5, 18, 19, 63–66, 141; lack of, 71

Orlikoff, James, 61

**P**

Pacific Business Group on Health, 92

Pain management, 132

Parkview Medical Center, Pueblo, Colorado, 32

Partnerships, between governing boards and CEOs, 67–78

Pathologists, exclusion from board membership, 57

Patient expectations, 84, 90

Patient harm. *See* Harm

Patient Protection and Affordable Care Act, 99

Patients, as quality committee members, 88

Patient safety, 96. *See also* Harm

Patient satisfaction, 85

Payments. *See also* Compensation: to board directors, 36–37, 38–39

Peer review, 80–81, 82, 90

Pennsylvania, business coalitions on health in, 93

Pennsylvania Hospital, 80

Performance evaluations. *See also* Self-assessments: of board chairs, 30; of board members, 12, 18, 151–155; of CEOs, 68, 69–70; by governance committees, 12; long version, sample of, 153–155; of new board members, 64; short version, sample of, 151–

152; versus term limits, 32–35

Personal interactions, between CEOs and board members, 73

Personnel costs, 116

Pet therapy, 133

Physicians: as board members, 55–61, 62; complementary and alternative medicine knowledge of, 133; decision making by, 59; hospital-based, 57

Piche, Gregory, 143–150

Planning committees, 12–13

Pneumonia, ventilator-associated, 83, 88

Pneumonia treatment, quality measurement of, 84–85

Policies, implementation of, 72

Population health. *See* Community health status

Poudre Valley Health System, Fort Collins, Colorado, 52

Premium revenues, 105

Premiums, in healthcare insurance, 99

Presbyterian Healthcare Services, Albuquerque, New Mexico, 61, 63

Preventive health programs, development of, 127

Primary care physicians, as board members, 58

Private hospitals, 501(c)(3) status of, 52

Process approach, to healthcare quality, 82–85

Profit, 106

Profitability ratios, 109, 112–113

Public Law 107-204. *See* Sarbanes-Oxley Act

**Q**

Quality, of healthcare: business case for, 88–89, 90; business coalitions and, 92–99; future issues in, 99–100; governing board's responsibility for, 3–4, 79–82, 90; history of, 79–82; process approach to, 82–85; systems approach to, 83–85; "three-legged stool" (Franklin) model of, 79–80

Quality and community health committees, 4, 13, 87–88, 126, 127–128

Quality assurance (QA), 81–82

Quality committees. *See* Quality and community healthcare committees

Quality improvement, strategies for, 85–88

importance of, 5–6; management's role in, 6–7

Strategic planning committees, 12–13

Stroke treatment, quality measurement of, 84–85

Structure, organizational: information about, 64; "three-legged stool" (Franklin) model of, 79–80

Succession planning, for chief executive officers (CEOs), 74–78

Surgery, Leapfrog Group's quality standards for, 97–98

Surgical sites, infection rate of, 82

Systems approach, to healthcare quality, 83–85

**T**

Tax-exempt status, 4; maintenance of, 9

Teamwork: among board members, 53, 59; obstacles to, 2

Tennessee, business coalitions on health in, 93

Terminology, of healthcare, 185–198; abbreviations and acronyms, 73, 182–185; of complementary and alternative medicine (CAM), 134–140

Term limits: for board chairs, 30; for board members, 31–35; disadvantages of, 32; versus performance evaluations, 32–35

Texas, business coalition on health in, 94

"Three-legged stool" (Franklin) model, 79–80

Time management, 1, 27

*To Err Is Human* (Institute of Medicine), 83, 96

Total asset turnover, 114–115

Tours, organizational, 65–66

Training, of board members, 55, 60

Transparency, 123, 128

*Trustee*, 5, 31, 55

Trustees. *See also* Board members: election of, 33

Turnover rate, of CEOs, 74–75

**U**

University of Colorado, 5, 34

**V**

Value-based purchasing, 89; by business coalitions for health, 94–95

Vanderbilt University Medical Center, Nashville, Tennessee, 61

Venous catheters, as infection cause, 83

Vice chairs, 20–21

Vice presidents, 3

Virginia, business coalition on health in, 94

Virginia Mason Medical Center, Seattle, Washington, 61, 63

Vision statements, 2–3; board members' commitment to, 54

Volunteers, as board members, 38, 39

**W**

Washington Business Group on Health, 92

Washington State, business coalitions on health in, 92, 94

Waste: measurement of, 98; reduction of, 99

Wilford, Dan, 62

Wisconsin, business coalition on health in, 94

Work plans, development of, 18

Wyoming, business coalition on health in, 94

**Y**

Yoga/yoga therapy, 132, 140

# About the Author

Errol L. Biggs, PhD, FACHE, is the director of the graduate programs in health administration and the director of the Center for Health Administration, University of Colorado Denver. Dr. Biggs received his PhD in health administration and planning from Pennsylvania State University, his LLB (law) degree from LaSalle Extension University, and an MBA in health administration from George Washington University.

Dr. Biggs's research and consulting activities include work with hospitals to improve the governance of those organizations. He teaches governance in both the graduate on-campus and executive programs in health administration at the University of Colorado. He is also a faculty member of Innovative Healthcare Speakers and the Center for Healthcare Governance and chairman of the Practical Governance Group, all of which offer educational programs for hospital governing boards.

Dr. Biggs has been involved in both the investor-owned and nonprofit hospital industries, including 12 years as the CEO of large teaching hospitals, and directed the first merger of an osteopathic (DO) hospital and an allopathic (MD) hospital in the United States.

Additionally, he has served on several nonprofit and investor-owned boards of directors. He conducts seminars and retreats for hospital boards of directors, and is the author of several articles on governance. In addition to this book, Dr. Biggs is also the coauthor of the popular book *Practical Governance*, published by Health Administration Press.

Dr. Biggs is a Fellow of the American College of Healthcare Executives. He is also a member of the National Association of Corporate Directors, BoardSource, the Association of University Programs in Health Administration, and the Medical Group Management Association.